THE PSYCHOLOGY OF SEX

What can psychology teach us about sex? How do different bodies and minds respond sexually? How can we prevent people being stigmatised for their sexuality?

The Psychology of Sex takes you on a tour through the different ways that psychologists have researched and theorised, and created and sustained, certain understandings of sex and sexuality. The book explores cultural concerns, such as sex and technology, trauma and consent, as well as drawing on research from sexual communities and the applied area of sex therapy.

When so much of our relationship to sex happens in the mind, *The Psychology of Sex* shows us how important it is to understand where our ideas about sex, and our erotic desires, come from.

Dr. Meg-John Barker is a writer and illustrator with a background in academic psychology, sex and relationship therapy, and queer activism. They've published a number of graphic guides and self-help style books on the themes of sex, gender, relationships and mental health, as well as free books and zines on topics such as trauma, consent and plurality. Website: rewriting-the-rules.com.

THE PSYCHOLOGY OF EVERYTHING

People are fascinated by psychology, and what makes humans tick. Why do we think and behave the way we do? We've all met arm-chair psychologists claiming to have the answers, and people that ask if psychologists can tell what they're thinking. *The Psychology of Everything* is a series of books which debunk the popular myths and pseudo-science surrounding some of life's biggest questions.

The series explores the hidden psychological factors that drive us, from our subconscious desires and aversions, to our natural social instincts. Absorbing, informative, and always intriguing, each book is written by an expert in the field, examining how research-based knowledge compares with popular wisdom, and showing how psychology can truly enrich our understanding of modern life.

Applying a psychological lens to an array of topics and contemporary concerns – from sex, to fashion, to conspiracy theories – *The Psychology of Everything* will make you look at everything in a new way.

Titles in the series:

The Psychology of Time by Richard Gross

The Psychology of Vaccination by Olivier Klein and Vincent Yzerbyt

The Psychology of Memory by Megan Sumeracki and Althea Need Kaminske

The Psychology of Artificial Intelligence by Tony J. Prescott

The Psychology of Trauma by Shanti Farrington and Alison Woodward

The Psychology of Menopause by Marie Percival

The Psychology of Fashion Second Edition by Carolyn Mair

The Psychology of the Extreme by Arie W. Kruglanski and Sophia Moskalenko

The Psychology of Stress by Charlotte Mottram, Alison Woodward, and Shanti Farrington

The Psychology of Sex by Meg-John Barker

For more information about this series, please visit: www.routledgetextbooks.com/textbooks/thepsychologyofeverything/

THE PSYCHOLOGY OF SEX

SECOND EDITION

MEG-JOHN BARKER

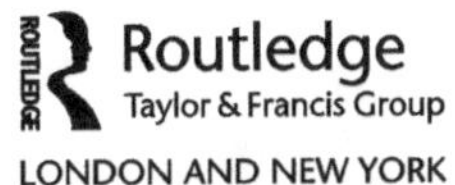

LONDON AND NEW YORK

Designed cover image: Routledge © Nigel Turner

Second edition published 2026
by Routledge
4 Park Square, Milton Park, Abingdon, Oxon, OX14 4RN

and by Routledge
605 Third Avenue, New York, NY 10158

Routledge is an imprint of the Taylor & Francis Group, an informa business

First edition published by Routledge 2018

British Library Cataloguing-in-Publication Data
A catalogue record for this book is available from the British Library

ISBN: 9781041217855 (hbk)
ISBN: 9781041217824 (pbk)
ISBN: 9781003728979 (ebk)

DOI: 10.4324/9781003728979

Typeset in Jonna
by codeMantra

CONTENTS

FOREWORD TO THE NEW EDITION

So much has happened in the world – and in all our lives – since the first edition of *The Psychology of Sex* was published back in 2018. It would be impossible to reflect all of this in a new edition. Instead I've focused on creating one major new chapter: on un/conscious sex. The rest of this book remains largely as it was, with a few points updated, and more recent references added in places. After an introduction to what's meant by 'psychology' and 'sex' (Chapter 1), the first four chapters of this book still deal with the history of how Western psychology – and the wider culture that informs it and is informed by it – came to understand sex and sexuality in the ways that it does and how this influences how we understand and experience sex ourselves.

Chapter 2 focuses on our sexualities, sexual orientations, or sexual identities and how they're frequently defined by who we're attracted to. Chapter 3 turns to sex acts and how notions of 'proper' sex, and functional and dysfunctional bodies, impact our erotic experiences. Chapter 4 explores sexual desires and how these have been categorised into 'normal' and 'abnormal' kinds, influencing how we feel about – and navigate – our erotic lives. Chapter 5 considers the kinds of debates that happen around sex, often as part of moral panics or culture wars. It explores how we might engage with these in a different way to polarising into two positions where one must be proved right and the other wrong, along with all the people who believe in it. For the second edition I've added some thoughts to this chapter about how we might think about sex and technology, given this is such a frequent focus of concern.

The new – final – chapter of this book deals with how our understandings of – and approaches to – sex, sexuality, and intimate relationships are often largely unconscious. It explores how becoming more conscious is vital, including increasing awareness of how we've been harmed – and can act in harmful ways – ourselves, both sexually and otherwise. Much of what plays out unconsciously are forms of cultural and personal trauma. Chapter 6 addresses how engaging consciously with the erotic might help us to become more trauma-aware, shame-sensitive, and connected in our relating (with ourselves, with others, within and between communities, and with the wider world): something that's urgently needed right now, in the arena of sex and in general.

Of course, a short book like this can only offer a very broad overview, and one which invariably oversimplifies things, telling one story when so many others could also have been told. Hopefully I've signposted enough places through the footnotes where you might go if you want to find out more, as well as giving you a sense of the kinds of questions we might helpfully ask about sex, and why continuing to ask them is so important.

If you'd like to explore your own sex and sexuality in more depth, I've written another book – with Alex Iantaffi – which provides tools about how to go about this.[1] That book includes a lot of material about how important it is to go slowly, and carefully, with ourselves when reading and reflecting on these topics. This is vital when so many of us have experienced sexual violence and non-consensual sexual experiences, and most of us have been harmed or constrained by prevailing views about sex and by sexual stigma and shame.

I'd invite you to go slowly and carefully with this book too, perhaps pausing to tune into yourself at the end of each section you read and stepping away if you feel at all overwhelmed or confused. There's more about how we might become more conscious and careful in our approach to sex at the end of Chapter 6, and all of that applies just as much to reading and talking about sex as it does to erotic activities. Feel free to read that part of the book first, or check out other resources about self-consent[2] before going on, especially if this is unfamiliar territory, or you have reasons for thinking this book will be particularly challenging for you.[3]

NOTES

1 Iantaffi, A., & Barker, M-J. (2021). *How to understand your sexuality*. Jessica Kingsley. See Further Resources for other suggested reading.

2 See artofconsent.co.uk/self-consent, loveuncommon.com/self-consent-courses

3 There are zines and other resources about practices for going slowly, tuning into our embodied feelings, and being consensual with ourselves on my website rewriting-the-rules.com, as well as at: loveuncommon.com, artofconsent.co.uk, schoolofconsent.org, and trueselftv.com.

1

PSYCHOLOGY AND SEX

Welcome to the psychology of sex. Like all of the books in *The Psychology of Everything* series, a short book like this can't give you a comprehensive overview of the whole of sex and sexuality from a psychological perspective. What it can do, though, is to give you a flavour of this area with the aim of whetting your appetite for more.

Also I hope that, above all else, you'll find this book *useful*. Like it or not we're all living in a world where we're constantly bombarded by sexual information, imagery, and ideologies. Psychology isn't just about finding things out with research, it's also about *evaluating* things psychologically and *applying* psychology to people's lives. So, in addition to giving you a lot of information about sex from various theories and studies, this book provides you with the tools to think *critically* about the messages you receive about sex and the debates you see playing out on sexual topics. It also includes a lot about how the psychological research and ideas can be *applied* to people's lives in general and also to your own life, relationships, and experiences.

Before we get started on specific topics in the psychology of sex, let's think a bit more broadly about these words we're using: 'psychology' and 'sex'. You might think it's obvious what they mean but actually they're both quite contested terms. In fact I hope that, throughout every chapter of this book, you'll continue to ask yourself

DOI: 10.4324/9781003728979-1

'what is psychology?' and 'what is sex?' and that the answers you give will change as you go along. As with many of the best questions there are no right answers to these ones, but rather it's important and useful to continually ask them and to notice how your answers shift as you reflect on them more.

WHAT IS PSYCHOLOGY?

The British Psychological Society, American Psychological Association, and other similar organisations tend to define psychology as something like 'the scientific study of mind and behaviour'.[1] From this we might understand psychology to be one amongst many scientific disciplines, in this case devoted to researching people's mental processes (mind) and how they act in the world (behaviour). The word 'scientific' might make us think of lab coats, experiments, and measuring these things in *objective* ways using numbers.

The narrow view

Certainly for much of its history psychology has been strongly invested in proving itself to be a science alongside other natural sciences like biology and physics. Students frequently choose a psychology degree because they're interested in people, would like to understand themselves better, or want to help people. So they're often surprised – and not always pleasantly so – by how much time they spend learning about mathematical statistics and brain processes!

A lot of the classic kinds of studies psychologists conduct do seem to support this fairly narrow definition of psychology as the science of mind and behaviour. For example, you might be familiar with the memory tests psychologists perform by flashing words up on a computer screen and measuring how many people can remember, examining whether the kind of word, or its place in the list, has an influence on how well it's remembered.[2] Or you may know about Stanley Milgram's classic studies on obedience, where he got people in a lab to think they were giving somebody gradually increasing electric shocks to help them learn, finding many people would give somebody a fatal electric shock if a person in a lab coat told them to do so.[3] Those are two examples of the scientific study of mind (memory) and behaviour (obedience to authority).

I worked in academic psychology for over twenty years. During that time I was part of several different psychology departments and had many different psychologist friends and colleagues. I learned from them that psychology is actually a good deal broader than what we might at first understand from a definition like 'the scientific study of mind and behaviour'.

The broad view

At its best I think psychology is the place where all the work which is relevant to our human experience comes together. It's a broad, encompassing discipline which draws together all of the knowledge we have which is relevant to people and which also looks outwards to address how we can improve people's lives. I have psychologist friends whose work is between psychology and history, psychology and geography, psychology and endocrinology, psychology and sociology, psychology and philosophy, psychology and neuroscience, psychology and criminology, psychology and drama, and many, many more. In fact I know of relatively few 'pure' psychologists. Most study psychology as it touches the edge of at least one other discipline (whether a natural science, a social science, or an arts or humanities subject).

Relatively few of these psychologists conduct lab experiments. Some are entirely engaged with developing theories, others study human behaviour in real-world settings, or interview people in-depth about their experiences, or study the history of psychological thinking, or use creative methods to help people produce something which is somewhere between research data and art. Most of them also apply psychological research and theories in some way, informing, for example, the worlds of law, medicine, social justice, counselling, media, or the environment. Some of them work entirely in an applied context, providing therapy, advising organisations, reducing crime, or helping kids in school, for example.

THE PSYCHOLOGY OF SEX

Turning to the subject of this book – or any of the other books in this series – you can see why this broad understanding of psychology is important.

Sex is a fascinating, far-reaching, and fraught area of human experience. We *could* limit ourselves to a narrow view of the psychology of sex and just focus on what we can learn about how people think and behave sexually, from experiments and questionnaires, for example. However, to really reach an understanding of how sex works, how people experience it, and what they think and feel about it, it's important to draw on knowledge from across a wide range of disciplines in conjunction with psychology.

We need to know the history of how people (including psychologists) have understood sex and sexuality and how that affects how we understand it today. We need to know about the physiology of sex and how different bodies and brains respond sexually. We need to look at sexual identities and practices across cultures and contexts and at the development of sexual communities and social movements. We need to draw on the wealth of theories that have developed in various branches of philosophy to understand sexuality and sexual relationships. We certainly need to bring the discipline of psychology together with biology and sociology, given that humans are embodied beings, entangled in relationships with others, and embedded in a cultural context,[4] all of which shapes how they think and behave sexually. And we absolutely need to study the work of the sexologists – people who have studied sex and sexuality specifically over the years – some but not all of whom are psychologists.

If the psychology of sex is going to be useful at all it also needs to speak to the urgent applied questions we have about sex: How can we stop people from being marginalised, stigmatised, or even tortured and killed for their sexuality? How can we help people who are struggling with sex? How can we reduce the frighteningly high rates of abusive and coercive sex? How can we help people who have survived sexual violence to heal and support those who have perpetrated such violence not to do it again? What would a healthy understanding of sex look like and how might we encourage the promotion of such an understanding in mainstream, social, and sexual media? How should we educate kids about sex? I'm sure you can think of many more.

Psychology is political

One debate which hasn't stopped raging in psychology since the 1970s is whether psychology can be neutral and objective or whether it's inevitably political: in other words, whether psychologists will have personal and cultural biases which influence what they study, how they study it, and what they find.

This is a vital issue for our purposes here because it influences how I write the rest of this book – and how you read it. Can I present you with a range of research findings and theories from psychology – in its broadest sense – so you can go away with the facts about the psychology of sex? Or will we both need to keep reminding ourselves about how all the studies and theories we're covering were produced by certain individuals in a certain time and place – perhaps seeing these findings and ideas as *one* way of understanding the psychology of sex but not as any kind of absolute fact?

Psychologists have often divided into two factions around these kinds of issues. The first faction we might call 'mainstream' psychologists (for want of a better word): those who believe it's possible for psychology to conduct objective value-free research to determine facts about human minds and behaviour. The second faction are often called 'critical' psychologists: those who believe psychological knowledge always develops in a certain specific situation which will affect what psychologists find and what they do with it. Critical psychologists are interested in how psychologists themselves *construct* knowledge in particular cultural contexts, rather than seeing psychological knowledge as a set of truths that can be uncovered. Knowledge could always have been built and shaped in alternative ways.

To overgeneralise quite a lot, mainstream psychologists have also tended to use *quantitative* research to *measure* human minds and behaviours in the form of numbers and to generalise their findings about the causes and effects of human behaviour to everybody. Critical psychologists have tended to use *qualitative* research to study how people talk about their *experience*, and they're often cautious not to generalise beyond the people they've studied directly. They're often more interested in *describing* experience than *explaining* it because they assume people's experience will vary according to their situation, cultural background, and so on.

In reality this binary mainstream/critical distinction is a false one, and thankfully it's breaking down over the years. Just as I struggled to find examples of colleagues who were entirely 'pure' or 'applied' psychologists, most of the more mainstream psychologists I know tend to be pretty critical in their thinking and recognise that personal and cultural biases always creep in when human beings are studying other human beings. And I also know a bunch of critical psychologists who use quantitative questions, lab experiments, and brain studies in their work. In this book I'll draw on work across this spectrum.

How psychology is shaped by individuals and their cultural context

A quick tour of the history of psychology shows us how impossible it is to study psychology in a completely objective way. Over and over again studies have found that even when they're trying to be completely unbiased, researchers will tend to find the results they expect to find. For example, if you give psychology trainees two groups of rats – or children – to study and tell them one group is more intelligent than the other, then that is exactly what they'll find, even when in actuality there's no difference between the two groups.[5] David Rosenhan's classic studies found that psychologists and psychiatrists would diagnose and treat somebody as mentally ill if they were in a mental health institution, even if they showed no signs of mental illness.[6] Clearly our expectations shape what we find in research and in professional psychological work.

The history of psychology also throws up some frankly terrifying examples of cultural biases influencing the work of psychologists. In his book *The Mismeasure of Man*,[7] Stephen J. Gould describes the project of intelligence testing to assess US army recruits in the First World War. Using the tests – which were regarded as highly scientifically rigorous – psychologists found the average intelligence of recruits decreased with the darkness of their skin, with Black people and immigrants to the US, including Jewish immigrants, obtaining the lowest scores. At the time, psychologists believed intelligence was entirely inherited, so the researchers concluded that different racial groups had different levels of 'natural' intelligence. These results were used as a basis for limiting immigration, due to fears of immigrants bringing down national intelligence. This prevented around six million Europeans from entering America between First World War and Second World War, condemning them to the Holocaust. The research also determined the ways army recruits were allocated, effectively condemning many Black soldiers to death.

When we look back on this intelligence research now, we recognise many biases which were not seen at the time because the research tallied so well with the prevailing cultural assumptions – in which the researchers were embedded. First, there were a lot of problems with the ways the research was conducted, meaning illiterate and foreign-born recruits were often given tests that required English literacy. Even when this didn't happen, they had to use a pencil, write numbers, and engage in other unfamiliar procedures. Also, many of the questions clearly did not test 'innate intellectual ability'. For example, there were pictures asking recruits to fill in the missing part of a lightbulb, gun, or playing card. And try answering these questions if you're not familiar with US culture: 'Crisco is a: patent medicine, disinfectant, toothpaste, food product?' 'Washington is to Adams as first is to . . .?' Indeed, the research found that foreign-born recruits did better depending on how many years they had been in the US, which should've given the researchers a clue that intelligence was not all down to 'nature'. We'll consider the nature/nurture debate in more depth in the next chapter.

In this example you can see how easy it is for psychologists to perpetuate and reinforce the prevailing views of the time: to divide people into categories on the basis of taken-for-granted knowledge without questioning it and then to find differences between those categories which they assume are down to innate differences between them, because that is widely held opinion, without looking hard enough for other explanations or examining the inbuilt biases in the materials they're using.

As Carol Tavris points out in her book *The Mismeasure of Women*,[8] there are many similar examples in the history of the psychology of gender. For example, early research on conformity found women were more likely to conform than men were. This was used to support the theory that women were naturally intellectually inferior to men. Later research found women and men are actually much the same when it comes to conformity, and whether we conform or not has far more to do with how much familiarity we have with the task we're given.[9] Early research had given people tasks that were more familiar to men than women because of the way they were brought up – for example, tasks about machinery. The psychologists then looked no further because the findings confirmed their misogynist assumptions.

You could conclude from these examples that psychologists in the past were biased but now we know so much more we could never make these kinds of mistakes. That would be a dangerous view as it would leave us much more open to making the same kinds of mistakes again. As psychologist Rosalind Gill so succinctly puts it, 'You can't step outside of culture', and we need to shine just as much a critical light on what we're doing now as we do on the past.[10]

The shaping of the psychology of sex

Certainly when I look across the psychology textbooks in the area of sex and sexuality it's very clear they're shaped by both prevailing cultural norms and the ways the particular psychologists involved situate themselves within those norms. The topics covered, the research and theories which writers deem important to include, and the ways these are discussed vary markedly from book to book.[11] I hope you'll think critically about the stories I'm telling about the psychology of sex here – just as you would with any other book. Like all authors I'm influenced by my own views and experience on this topic and my cultural context and how I relate to it.[12]

My plan in this book is to tell you about what psychology has discovered about sex and sexuality and also about how psychology itself has been involved in creating and sustaining certain understandings of sex and sexuality. It's important for you to hold in mind the fact that it does both of these things. In Chapter 2 we'll see that the ways psychologists and sexologists have measured sexuality have been influenced by prevailing cultural understandings of sexuality as well as contributing to those very understandings. In Chapters 3 and 4 we'll see how the diagnostic categories of sexual problems and 'paraphilias' used by psychiatrists and psychologists have changed dramatically over the years: clear evidence of the relationship between psychology and the shifting culture in which it lives. In Chapter 5 we'll explore research and theories produced by psychologists on the different sides of current debates around sex and sexuality. In Chapter 6 we'll consider how collective and personal experiences – particularly trauma – massively impact all of our unconscious processes around sex and sexuality, including psychologists of course.

WHAT IS SEX?

This is the question we'll continually ask over the course of this book as we explore the psychological theories and research in this area, both in terms of what they've contributed to our knowledge about sex and how they've bolstered or challenged prevailing cultural assumptions.

As with many topics relating to the psychology of everyday life, sex is something many people *think* they already know about, from their own experience and from the ideas about sex which circulate in our culture and tend to be taken as fact. For many of the topics in this book I'll start with this 'common sense' knowledge. What are the taken-for-granteds when people talk about sex or the popular ideas in sex advice, TV shows, or online forums? Then I'll unpack the psychological theories and research in the area to examine the evidence for our common sense views and to explore the ways psychology – and other related academic disciplines – have contributed to our current understandings of sex.

Sex is also a curious topic because it's simultaneously everywhere and nowhere. As you'll see in Chapter 5, there's often a sense that we're living in a world saturated with sexual images and messages, advice, and warnings. It's very easy – at the click of a button – to access videos of people having sex, information about any sexual practice or problem, and all kinds of opinions about the latest sex scandal. But at the same time, sex remains hugely taboo. Over the course of this book you'll see there's still a lot of anxiety about stepping outside the sexual norm, fear around measuring up sexually and being sexy enough, and deep concern around sexual violence and non-consent. People don't communicate about sex with health professionals, with their kids, or even with the people they're actually having sex with. People are still ridiculed, stigmatised, marginalised, pathologised, and criminalised on the basis of their sexual practices and preferences. People struggle to tune in to what they want sexually and to convey that to others, making consent very challenging.

For these reasons it's particularly important that psychologists – and other academics and professionals – obtain and promote clear, accurate, and helpful information about sex. It's also vital that they recognise the ways their theories and research will be *influenced by* their own experiences and the culture they operate within, as well as the power they have to *shape* that culture and other people's experiences (and the responsibility which goes along with this power).[13]

To summarise what we've covered in this chapter, the following diagram illustrates the potential interrelationships between psychology, popular culture, and individual experiences in this area (Figure 1.1).

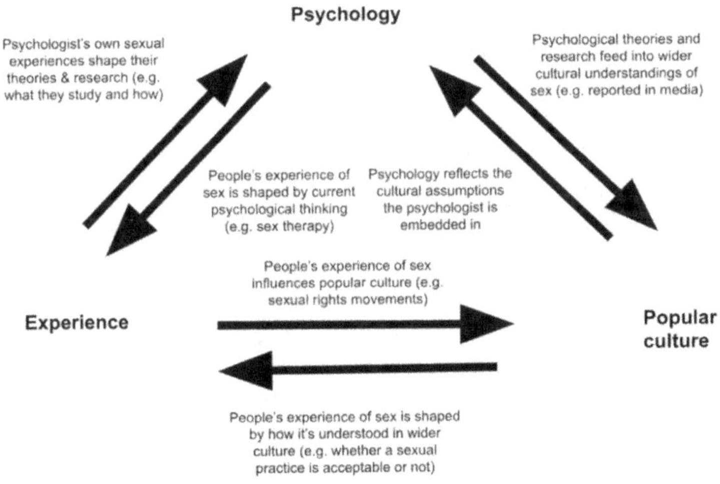

FIGURE 1.1 Psychology, popular culture, and individual experience

HOW TO READ THIS BOOK

You might find it helpful to return to this diagram a few times while you read the rest of this book because we'll explore several examples of the various processes summarised here. Many of the examples are historical – because it's often easier to see how such things have happened in the past – but it's vital to keep remembering they equally apply to the psychology of sex we're involved in today. In a hundred years' time the work psychologists are doing now may well look just as strange and disturbing to people reading about it as the intelligence testing and gender conformity examples mentioned in this chapter do to us now.

Over the next five chapters we'll consider five different meanings of sex:

- Chapter 2: Sex in the context of sexuality or sexual orientation, and sex meaning gender (the sex you're attracted to).
- Chapter 3: Sex as in 'the sex act' or 'sexual intercourse' and what is considered functional and dysfunctional sex.
- Chapter 4: Sex as in sexual practices and sexual relationships, and which are defined as normal or abnormal.
- Chapter 5: Sex as in sexiness, 'great sex', and concerns around people becoming 'sexualised'.
- Chapter 6: Sex as in the erotic, unconscious processes, and sexual trauma.

NOTES

1 When I'm talking about psychology I'm generally referring to Western psychology within a Western cultural context. While this book focuses mainly on how Western psychology has understood sex and sexuality and the impact this has had, there's huge scope for engaging further with psychologies that have developed in other cultural contexts as well as with the vast cultural diversity which exists in understandings of sex and sexuality. We'll touch on the issues with our understandings of sex being embedded in a Western capitalist, colonialist context in Chapter 6. For more on global understandings and experiences of sexuality see: Davy, Z., Thoreson, R., Bertone, C., & Santos, A. C. (2020). *The SAGE handbook of global sexualities*. Sage.

2 There's a nice overview of some of these studies here: simplypsychology.org/primacy-recency.html

3 You can read about this study, and some reflections on it here: theatlantic.com/health/archive/2015/01/rethinking-one-of-psychologys-most-infamous-experiments/384913

4 See the Queer Creative Health 1 and 2 zines for more on this under standing, and how it relates to research: rewriting-the-rules.com/zines.

5 You can read about Robert Rosenthal's work on expectancy effects – which include these studies – as well as many more examples of how both psychologists and participants behave differently when they're involved in psychological studies here: psy.gla.ac.uk/~steve/hawth.html

6 Rosenhan, D. L. (1973). On being sane in insane places. *Science*, *179*, 250–258. An updated version of this study is reported in Slater, L. (2004). *Opening Skinner's box: Great psychological experiments of the twentieth century*. W. W. Norton.

7 Gould, S. J. (1996). *The mismeasure of man*. W. W. Norton.

8 Tavris, C. (1991). *The mismeasure of woman: Paradoxes and perspectives in the study of gender*. American Psychological Association.

9 Sistrunk, F., & McDavid, J. W. (1971). Sex variable in conforming behaviour. *Journal of Personality and Social Psychology*, *2*, 200–207.

10 For more on how Western psychology has been shaped by history and culture and how we need to keep attending to these issues, an excellent book is: Jones, D., & Elcock, J. (2001). *History and theories of psychology: A critical perspective*. Arnold. A more recent example demonstrating how psychologists still use their research to endorse problematic practices because of prevailing cultural understandings is the involvement of eminent psychologists in the torture of detainees: economist.com/blogs/democracyinamerica/2015/07/terror-torture-and-psychology

11 You might like to compare, for example, the contents pages of Justin Lehmiller's *The psychology of human sexuality* (Blackwell, 2023), Chess Denman's *Sexuality: A biopsychosocial approach* (Palgrave, 2017), and Ann Bolin and colleagues' *Human sexuality: Biological, psychological, and cultural perspectives* (Routledge, 2021). You'd see even more variation if you looked back over the content pages of psychology of sexuality textbooks from the last century.

12 You can read more about what these are in Iantaffi, A., & Barker, M-J. (2021). *How to understand your sexuality*. Jessica Kingsley.

13 Spiderman (timeless).

2

SEX AND SEXUALITY

We tend to see sex as a fundamental aspect of who we are as human beings. A person's *sexuality* is regarded as a vital aspect of their identity: a key piece of demographic information to measure alongside their gender, age, and ethnicity. We think it's important for people to be open about their sexuality: to 'come out' about who they are. And our knowledge or assumptions about a person's sexuality affect our expectations about what they'll be like as a person.

WHAT IS SEXUALITY?

But what do we mean by sexuality? Think for a moment about what your answer would be if you were asked for your sexuality on a form or questionnaire.

Before we get into this chapter let's pull out some of the common cultural assumptions about sexuality. As we do so, you can start to think about whether or not they reflect your understanding and experience of sexuality.

The terms 'sexuality', 'sexual identity', and 'sexual orientation' tend to be used fairly interchangeably, and the latter two terms help to unpack what we generally mean by sexuality. It's a key feature of

DOI: 10.4324/9781003728979-2

a person's identity which is defined by who they *orient* towards sexually: in other words, who they're sexually attracted to.

As an *identity*, sexuality is generally assumed to be an *essential* aspect of who we are: part of our fundamental essence as a human being. As such, it's expected to be fixed and unchanging over the course of a life, which is partly why it makes sense to ask it as a piece of demographic information. It's often assumed to be a natural or biological feature of who we are: you were born this way and you'll stay this way.

As an *orientation*, sexuality is all about who we're sexually attracted to in terms of our sex and theirs. Are we attracted to the 'opposite sex' or the 'same sex'? Are we heterosexual or homosexual? There's generally an assumption that people are heterosexual unless they say otherwise. Coming out is associated with gay rather than straight people. Also we tend to ask more questions of people who aren't heterosexual (when did you realise? how do you know? why are you?), suggesting we generally view heterosexuality as the norm and homosexuality as something other (Table 2.1).

TABLE 2.1 Sexual orientation

		Attracted to	
		Male	*Female*
Person is	**Male**	Homosexual	Heterosexual
	Female	Heterosexual	Homosexual

So, to summarise the common cultural understanding of sexuality:

- Sexuality is *binary* (you're either heterosexual or you're homosexual).
- Sexuality is an aspect of identity whereby we can *categorise* people into one of these two boxes.
- Sexuality is *essential*: a feature of who we are which is fixed and unchanging over time.

- Sexuality is all about our sex and the sex of people we're attracted to (whether we're male or female and whether we're attracted to males or females).
- Sexuality is a *natural* feature of who we are: something we're born with.

PSYCHOLOGY AND SEXUALITY

These ideas about sexuality may seem obvious: just something many of us take for granted. However, reading down the list you'll probably have already started to question some of them. You might have thought 'Hang on, what about bisexuality?' or 'I know someone whose sexuality changed in later life', or 'Isn't there a debate about whether it's nature or nurture?'

You'll see in this chapter that psychology has had a major role over the last 150 years or so in shaping these ideas and in cementing them in the public consciousness. More recently, however, psychologists have also been involved in questioning these assumptions and in conducting research finding that sexuality may be a good deal more diverse and complex than this common set of understandings would suggest.

The rest of this chapter takes you through different ways psychologists – and other scientists and social scientists – have *measured* sexuality. This will help you to explore each of these assumptions further. It's also a helpful way of demonstrating that the ways psychologists define and measure things aren't completely neutral and objective (as we touched on in Chapter 1). Rather, definitions and measurements are often rooted in the wider cultural assumptions which psychologists – as human beings within that culture – tend to accept. Research based on these measures often then reinforces these assumptions.

GAY OR STRAIGHT?

The first time most of us were called upon to think about our sexuality, it was probably framed in this way: 'Are you straight or are you gay?' Up until the point we found out about these possibilities it's quite likely we'll have assumed that we – and other people – would be heterosexual, given that the overwhelming majority of books, movies, and teaching materials aimed at kids represent male/female couples and families with mothers and fathers.[1] Just think about the stories, kids' films, and lessons you remember from when you were growing up. This assumption that people are straight is called *heteronormativity*.

Sadly, most people still learn about the possibility of being something other than straight in the context of that alternative being a negative (or at least strange) thing. The word 'gay' and derogatory terms for homosexuality remain popular playground insults.[2]

This idea that people are heterosexual or homosexual isn't how people have always understood sexuality, though. Historians of sexuality talk about 'the invention of homosexuality' in the nineteenth century. If you'd lived before that time it wouldn't have made sense to you to think of a person as gay – or as straight either.

Early sexology

Towards the end of the nineteenth century various scholars began the project of classifying and categorising sex. At that point psychology was still in its infancy, and many of the early sexologists were psychiatrists or other kinds of medics rather than psychologists as such. Sexologists such as Richard von Krafft-Ebing, Magnus Hirschfeld, and Henry Havelock Ellis applied the approach of classification which was popular in medicine and science to the field of sexuality. Generally they attempted to categorise different types of sexual deviance.

We'll return to the importance of early sexology in shaping our thinking about sex in terms of normality and abnormality in Chapter 4. What's important for our purposes here is that these classifications started a shift from sexuality being seen as something you *did* to something you *were*. Before that time some sexual behaviours – such as sodomy – had been regarded as a sin or a crime but not as something that made you a certain type of person. That's why we can talk about the 'invention' of homosexuality – and heterosexuality. Before that time a person wouldn't have been seen as a homosexual or as a heterosexual.

This understanding of sexuality as an identity had a marked impact on how people have been treated ever since. It meant people could now be discriminated against, criminalised, and pathologised on the basis of their sexuality: being seen as a fundamentally bad, wrong, or sick kind of person. It also meant people could fight for rights; their sexuality made them a certain kind of person who should be treated equally to everyone else. Indeed, some of the first sexologists were involved in the earliest versions of the gay rights movement.

Freud and psychoanalysis

The famous father of psychoanalysis, Sigmund Freud, was responsible for developing the ideas of the early sexologists and planting them clearly in the popular imagination. While most of the early sexologists believed there were biomedical explanations for a person's sexuality, Freud believed sexuality was something that developed over time. Freud was still *essentialist*, however, because he saw sexuality as a fundamental feature of who a person was which was fixed by the time they became an adult.

Freud believed there were two key aspects of sexuality: the sexual *aim* and the sexual *object*. We'll return to the sexual aim in the next chapter because that's about the parts of the body we get sexual satisfaction from.

Freud's theory of the sexual object was vital for setting in stone the gay/straight binary we're exploring here. His theory held that people were born 'polymorphously perverse' and capable of attraction regardless of a person's gender. However, through a set of developmental stages they came to a mature sexuality. Freud theorised that people reach a stable sexual *object choice*: attraction to the opposite sex after going through the Oedipus complex. This involves coming to identify with the same-sex parent after having previously desired their opposite-sex parent and seen the same-sex parent as a rival. Not going through the Oedipus complex fully could leave someone attracted to the same sex.

So we can see that the early sexologists and psychoanalysts set the blueprint for how we think about sexuality today: as a fundamental aspect of our identity and as a binary: being attracted to the same or opposite sex.

Psychology and the straight/gay binary

Most mainstream psychologists today are fairly critical of Freud's theories.[3] However, the idea that people have an inherent sexual orientation towards the same or opposite sex has remained relatively unchallenged.

While I was an academic psychologist, I reviewed the main psychology textbooks of the time to see how they covered sexuality.[4] I found this topic was almost exclusively covered in the biological psychology sections of textbooks – and indeed the dominant way of understanding sexuality has definitely swung back from nurture to nature since Freud's day. Most of the textbooks covered sexuality in the same way: in a section covering (mostly biological) explanations for why some people are gay. Particularly common was the search for the 'gay gene' and associated research on differences between straight and gay people which might suggest a genetic cause. We'll touch on this again later when we return to the nature/nurture question.

Such analyses suggest it's still common in psychology to regard sexuality as fixed and binary, with heterosexuality being the assumed norm and homosexuality therefore requiring some kind of explanation for its existence.[5]

Invisible bisexuals in psychology

Importantly, for what we're thinking about here, I found very little mention of the possibility of bisexuality in psychology textbooks.

Half didn't acknowledge its existence at all, asking questions like 'Why do some people prefer partners of the other sex and some prefer partners of their own sex?' with no recognition that some might prefer either or both. The other half of the books touched on bisexuality very briefly and then went on to cover only theories and research relating to straight and gay people. Often these mentions of bisexuality happened in order to downplay it: either arguing that it didn't exist at all or that it was extremely rare.

This questioning of bisexuality as a legitimate sexual orientation has been common in psychology. Many psychologists have insisted that sexuality is binary and therefore bisexuality cannot exist.

One particularly famous study was reported in the *New York Times* as proving bisexual men were 'straight, gay, or lying'.[6] It claimed to have found that men who identified as bisexual actually responded only in a 'homosexual' or 'heterosexual' manner.[7] In this study men who identified as gay, straight, or bisexual were wired up to a *penile plethysmograph* device, which measures the extent of erection in the penis. They were then shown pornographic films of two men having sex or two women having sex. Around a third of the participants didn't respond sufficiently to either stimulus to be included in the data analysis. Of those remaining they generally responded either to the first movie or to the second, but not to both. You might want to pause for a moment to consider what you think of this study. Is measuring physiological arousal a good way at getting at a person's 'true' sexual orientation? Do you agree it supports the conclusion that bisexual attraction doesn't exist?

The study was criticised for several reasons. Certainly we might question whether people are 'homosexually attracted' if their penises respond to images of two men having sex and 'heterosexually attracted' if their penises respond to images of two women having sex. Obviously the researchers wanted to avoid having pornography with a man and a woman in it because the results would be unclear, but are all heterosexual men attracted to two women together? Would we conclude that a woman was heterosexual if she responded to a film of two men together? Also it seems possible that many bisexual men may well have been excluded from the study as part of the group who didn't show sufficient arousal to either film to be included.

Interestingly the study was repeated by the same research laboratory a few years later.[8] After taking on board the criticisms, the lab *did* then find participants who showed a pattern of bisexual attraction. This represents a wider shift in psychology towards acknowledging the existence of bisexuality, although there is still slow progress in breaking down binary assumptions.[9]

Culturally the binary understanding of sexuality seems very embedded,[10] and bisexuality is still frequently represented in the media as questionable, suspicious, 'just a phase', or not existing at all. Psychological research on mental health which does tease out bisexual experience overwhelmingly finds that bisexual people experience worse mental health than heterosexual or lesbian and gay people. This has been linked to the fact that bisexual people are frequently denied or stigmatised because of their sexuality.[11] We might ask ourselves what it was like to live as a bisexual man in the years between the original study and the repeated version, when it was commonly held that science had proved he was really gay, straight, or lying.

CATEGORIES OR CONTINUUM?

So we've seen there's generally agreement in psychology these days that sexuality isn't binary, and this is slowly filtering into popular culture. For this reason, studies of sexuality – like the ones I just mentioned on mental health – would tend to now include a demographic scale including at least *three* categories for sexuality. To see what this might look like, here's the demographic scale of sexual orientation used on the UK census at the time of writing.[12]

Demographic categories

Which of the following options best describes how you think of yourself?

Heterosexual or straight □
Gay or lesbian □
Bisexual □
Other sexual orientation □
(Write in sexual orientation)

You might like to pause and think for yourself which box you'd tick here. What kind of demographic data does it capture, and what's missing from it, in relation to understanding a person's sexuality?

In answer to this question you might have considered that these sexual orientation labels give us a good sense of how a person defines themselves but not necessarily much of a sense of this person's actual behaviours or attractions. This is one of the issues penile plethysmography and vaginal photoplethysmography studies are attempting to address. For example, somebody might have had sexual experiences or attractions to more than one gender but still label themselves as straight or gay, perhaps because they're worried about homophobia (if they identify as straight) or because they feel they're part of a gay community (if they identify as gay) and don't want to be rejected by that community.

The idea of identifying yourself as a certain sexual orientation is also culturally specific: not all cultures and communities do this. Finally, there are only three named options here: heterosexual, bisexual, or gay. You might wonder whether that covers the full diversity of people's possible sexual attractions. We'll come back to this shortly.

So what other ways might there be of measuring a person's sexuality if we recognise identity labels don't completely capture it? One example you've probably heard of is the Kinsey scale. This takes the recognition that sexuality isn't binary a stage further than adding an additional category of bisexual between homosexual and heterosexual: it imagines sexuality on a spectrum or continuum.

Alfred Kinsey was a biologist working in the US in the 1940s. He noticed the negative impact the massive cultural taboos and ignorance around sex at the time had on him and on the students he taught. Some of this was a legacy of the sexologies of deviance and psychoanalytic theories we touched on earlier. For this reason Kinsey set out to study sex scientifically: to inform everyone about what people were really doing sexually. Two books were published based on his team's extensive sex history interviews with thousands of people, *Sexual Behavior in the Human Male* and *Sexual Behavior in the Human Female*. These are popularly known as the Kinsey Reports and became instant bestsellers.[13] Amongst other findings which shook cultural assumptions about sex to their foundations, the Kinsey research found that 92% of men and 62% of women had masturbated, 70% of couples engaged in oral sex and 11% anal sex, and between 67% and 98% of men and around 50% of women had had sex before marriage.[14]

What is of most interest to us here, though, is the Kinsey scale. Because Kinsey was interested in behaviour rather than identity, instead of asking people their sexuality he placed them on a continuum from exclusively heterosexual to exclusively homosexual on the basis of their sexual experience.

The Kinsey scale

- 0 exclusively heterosexual
- 1 predominantly heterosexual, only incidentally homosexual
- 2 predominantly heterosexual but more than incidentally homosexual
- 3 equally heterosexual and homosexual
- 4 predominantly homosexual but more than incidentally heterosexual
- 5 predominantly homosexual, only incidentally heterosexual
- 6 exclusively homosexual
- X No sexual attraction

On the basis of this, Kinsey found that 2–6% of women and 4% of men were exclusively homosexual. A range of 6–14% of women and 46% of men had had both heterosexual and homosexual experiences and 13% of women and 37% of men had had at least one homosexual experience to the point of orgasm.

Pause for a moment and consider where you'd fall on the Kinsey scale. Did you have any trouble deciding? What do you think the Kinsey scale captures and what's missing from it, in relation to understanding a person's sexuality?

The Kinsey scale is based on experience rather than identity, and it gets at a range of experiences. This is important because we get very different statistics when we ask about sexual identity to when we ask about sexual experience. Looking across all of the US and UK studies, over three times as many people say they've had at least one same-sex sexual experience as those who identify as lesbian, gay, or bisexual (LGB). In the most recent UK example, at the time of writing, the surveying company YouGov found that 7% of adults identified as LGBTQ+.[15] When they were asked to place themselves on the Kinsey scale, however, 67% of all adults and 46% of adults aged 18–24 years put themselves at zero; 2% of all adults and 6% of young adults put themselves at six.[16] That means a quarter of all adults and half of young adults placed themselves somewhere between the extremes. This is a fascinating statistic to consider alongside the long-held cultural and psychological view that bisexuality doesn't exist or is extremely rare.

Kinsey's research has been criticised for how the data were collected and analysed – which makes it difficult to tell whether the findings were representative of the whole population. Again, this alerts us to the fact that the ways psychologists – and other scientists – study sex and sexuality have a marked impact on what they find. The shifting numbers over the years, across different studies, cultures, and generations, also suggest there is some social element to how we experience, identify, and report on our sexuality – something we'll return to towards the end of this chapter.[17]

While Kinsey's findings were based on people's reported sexual behaviour, it isn't completely clear whether the YouGov survey respondents are talking about their experience or their attractions. This diagram helps us to think about how the proportions are likely to differ depending on the question we're asking (Figure 2.1).

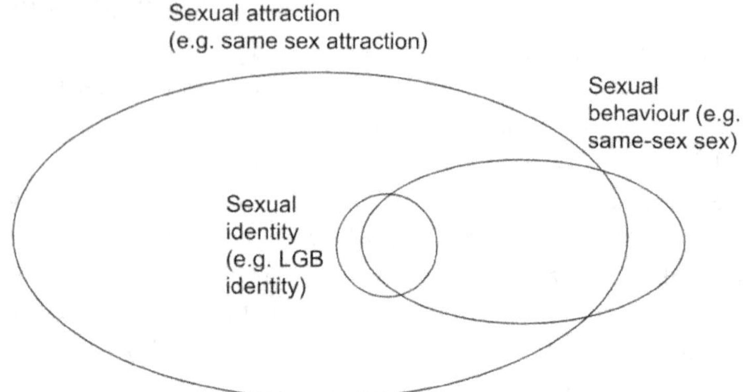

FIGURE 2.1 Sexual identity, behaviour, and attraction

Identity, experience, attraction

For any aspect of sexuality the greatest proportion of people are likely to have that attraction without necessarily acting on it or identifying with it. A smaller subset will behave in that way, and a smaller subset will identify that way. The overlaps on the diagram are because some people will identify with a sexuality without necessarily having acted upon it (young people and celibate people, for example), and some people will sometimes behave in a way which doesn't match their sexual attraction (some actors, sex workers, and people learning about their sexuality, for example).

Another drawback of the Kinsey scale – at least as it was used in the YouGov survey – is that, like demographic identity terms, it only gives us a snapshot of how somebody sees their sexuality at the point in time they're completing the survey. Therefore, if we're not careful, research like this – which takes place at one point in time and relies on a single measure – can give the impression sexuality is a relatively static, fixed thing – without actually checking whether that is the case.

FIXED OR FLUID?

Fritz Klein, a US sexologist and psychiatrist who followed Kinsey, came up with this grid for studying sexuality, due to the problems I

TABLE 2.2 The Klein grid

	Terms	More than 10 years ago	More than 5 years ago	More than a year ago	In the past year	In the future
1	Sexual attraction – who turns you on					
2	Sexual behaviour – who you have sex with					
3	Sexual fantasies – who you have sexual fantasies about					
4	Emotional preference – who you have strong emotional bonds with					
5	Social preference – who you like to spend your leisure time with					
6	Lifestyle – the sexual identity of the people you spend time with					
7	Sexual identity – how you self identify					
8	Political identify – who you identify with					

Scale used for rows 1–5: 1 = Other sex only, 2 = Other sex mostly, 3 = Other sex somewhat more, 4 = Both sexes equally, 5 = Same sex somewhat more, 6 = Same sex mostly, 7 = Same sex only, 0 = Does not apply

Scale used for rows 6–8: 1 = Heterosexual only, 2 = Heterosexual mostly, 3 = Bisexual mostly, some hetero, 4 = Bisexual only, 5 = Bisexual mostly some homo, 6 = Homosexual mostly, 7 = Homosexual only

just mentioned with the Kinsey scale.[18] You might like to have a go at filling it in yourself, or just think about whether it's a better or worse measure than Kinsey's (Table 2.2).

You might notice this scale gets at sexual attraction, behaviour, *and* identity, rather than only studying one of these. It also captures some additional dimensions to sexuality, such as political identity, which may differ from sexual identity. For example, somebody could be very involved in LGB rights without necessarily being LGB themselves, perhaps due to friends or family members being LGB. It also builds in the important possibility that all of these aspects might change over time, rather than regarding sexual experience or identity as fixed and static. Research using this grid has found that the numbers people give for each dimension often do vary across time.[19]

Sexual fluidity

Klein's theory that sexuality could be dynamic did not catch on immediately when he was writing about these matters in the 1980s, and certainly the Klein grid never gained the kind of popular attention the Kinsey scale has received. Recent years, however, have seen renewed attention to the concept of dynamic sexuality or *sexual fluidity*. A key researcher in this area is Lisa Diamond.[20] Diamond studied a hundred women who experienced some degree of same-sex attraction over the course of a decade. She found that around two-thirds of the women changed their sexual identity label at least once during this period and in all possible directions (lesbian to bisexual, bisexual to heterosexual, unlabelled to lesbian, etc.). These changes often coincided with the gender of their current sexual or romantic partners. Diamond concluded that this demonstrated sexual fluidity: the capacity to adapt sexual and romantic attraction to a specific person instead of to an overall gender category.

Since Diamond's initial study there has been a lot of focus on gender differences in sexual fluidity, with many psychologists suggesting women are more sexually fluid than men. For example, going back to the physiological arousal studies I mentioned earlier, Meredith Chivers and colleagues found that women tended to respond genitally to all kinds of depictions of sex acts (including those between men and women, between women, and between animals), whereas men responded more specifically depending on the gender of the people they were watching (in line with their sexual orientation).[21] Like Diamond, Ritch Savin Williams and his colleagues conducted a study of sexual identity over time and found that men's identity labels were less likely to change than women's.[22] However, another national US survey found that half of men with a bisexual identity showed identity change over time, so being male doesn't necessarily mean having a rigid or fixed sexuality.[23]

While some researchers argue for some fundamental gender difference to explain these kinds of findings, it's also important to consider the role of cultural homophobia and biphobia here. Masculinity is still strongly defined against femininity and homosexuality in much of society:[24] being a 'real man' means not being feminine and not being gay. In support of cultural involvement, another study of men who had sex with men found that more of them identified as straight than gay, and almost none as bisexual.[25] Whatever the reason, it seems clear that some people experience their sexuality as relatively fixed over time and some as rather more fluid and changeable.[26]

You might find it helpful to reflect on which aspects of your sexuality, and which kinds of people you find attractive (if any), have changed over time and which have stayed relatively stable. It's important to emphasise here that sexual fluidity doesn't equate to 'changeable at will'. While some people have found that different sexual experiences open up attractions and arousal patterns they hadn't realised were possible, endeavours to change a person's sexuality – usually to conform to a more culturally acceptable pattern – have overwhelmingly failed and are ethically very highly questionable.[27]

ALL ABOUT SEX?

There's one more thing you might have noticed across all the research we've explored here so far, whether it used demographic lists, or continuums, or physiological arousal measures. In fact you might *not* have noticed it because it's taken for granted by most psychologists. This is the assumption that sexuality – whether identity, experience, or attraction and whether fixed or fluid – is all about the sex of the person we're attracted to. Even the Kinsey scale and the Klein grid assume that the defining feature of a person's sexuality is the extent to which they're attracted to the same sex or the opposite sex.

There are two issues with this. First, like sexual orientation, sex and gender are not binary, so the 'same or opposite' distinction we've been using is problematic. Second, it fails to account for all of the other features of a person's sexuality which might be as important as or even more important than the sex or gender of the people they find attractive or have sex with.

Sex/gender

Psychologists often use the word 'sex' to refer to our biological features and gender to refer to whether somebody takes on the roles and behaviours which are socially associated with masculinity or femininity (or both or neither). Actually it's a lot more complex than this because there are a whole lot of different aspects of our biological, psychological, and social sex/gender, and none of these are simply binary (male or female).

Starting with biology, there's diversity across all levels of sex/gender. There is diversity in chromosomal makeup, in hormonal sensitivity and take-up, and in genitals (so it's not always clear what is a penis or a clitoris). There's also diversity in all of the physical aspects which we tend to regard as 'male' or' female', with many people fitting better on the 'opposite' end of the spectrum than we might predict by gender stereotypes (e.g. in terms of height, voice pitch, strength, hairiness, and chest size). As geneticist Anne Fausto-Sterling puts it:

> While male and female stand on the extreme ends of a biological continuum, there are many bodies . . . that evidently mix together anatomical components conventionally attributed to both males and females. . . . Modern surgical techniques help maintain the two-sex system. Today children who are born 'either/or–neither/both' – a fairly common phenomenon – usually disappear from view because doctors 'correct' them right away with surgery.[28]

Research has found that brains too are not binary. Neuroscientist Daphna Joel and colleagues found that the idea of the 'male' and 'female' brain is a myth: between 0 and 8% of people have all of the brain features they might be expected to have, based on their sex. The vast majority of people have some combination of these features.[29] Another neuroscientist, Cordelia Fine, has also emphasised *neuroplasticity*: the fact many of the gender differences that *are* found in the brain are due to the way people have learnt gender roles – meaning certain neural connections have been made and not others.[30] Gendered brain differences are often a product of gender experience, rather than a cause of it.

It's not surprising, then, that globally many cultures recognise more than two genders.[31] Despite the tendency in the west to view gender as binary, as with sexuality things seem to be starting to shift here too. You might be familiar with the range of over 70 gender identity terms that Facebook offers including options such as bigender, gender neutral, androgynous, genderqueer, and gender fluid. According to official statistics, the proportion of the UK population who define as non-binary when given an option beyond male and female is between 1 in 1700 and 1 in 250 people.[32] However, in another study by Daphna Joel and colleagues, they found that, in a general population, over a third of people said they were to some extent the 'other' gender, 'both genders', and/or 'neither gender'.[33]

You might pause and think to yourself whether you, or the people you know, fit perfectly into the cultural stereotypes of masculinity or femininity.[34]

As with sexuality, some people experience their gender as very fixed, some as fluid and changing, and everything in between. For some (cisgender) people the gender they're assigned at birth – generally on the basis of their genitalia – fits their experience of their gender, for other (trans) people – including non-binary people – it does not.

Going back to the diagram of our cultural understanding of sexual orientation earlier in this chapter, you saw how it assumes both sexuality and gender to be binary (male/female, gay/straight), but perhaps these binary categories have been imposed on a human experience that isn't binary at all. If that's the case then any measure of sexuality that assumes there are two, and only two, genders that a person could be attracted to (same, opposite, or some degree of both) is going to be flawed.

Focus on sex/gender of attraction

There's another, perhaps even more significant, problem here: the importance placed on both gender and sexual orientation in defining a person. Psychologist Sandra Bem raised the question of why gender is seen as such an important feature throughout her work. She argued that gender was not useful as an organising category and that psychology – and wider culture – should move away from the use of gender categories entirely.[35] The same could be said for sexual orientation. If you remember back to Lisa Diamond's work, she found that for many of the women she studied, their sexuality was much more about the person they found attractive, or had a relationship with, than their gender.

This accords with research on bisexual and pansexual people which has found that many define these terms as being attracted to people 'regardless of gender', seeing gender as a feature of potential partners no more important than eye colour, for example.[36] It also makes sense of the way sexual identity terms have exploded in recent years – in a similar way to the gender terms on Facebook. Younger people are increasingly using multiple terms to describe their sexuality, including kinky, polyamarous, asexual, abrosexual, sapiosexual, skoliosexual, and many other terms.[37]

Some psychologists – and other social scientists – study sexuality more *qualitatively* than *quantitatively*: asking people with certain sexualities to describe or discuss their experience, rather than trying to capture it in numbers. They often find there is little focus on gender of attraction when you approach it in this way. Rather, people talk in much more depth about other aspects related to their sexuality: such as their sense of belonging to a social group and ability to 'be themselves',[38] or the rich detail of their specific sexual fantasies and experiences.[39]

Sexuality theorist Eve Kosofsky Sedgwick comments on the narrow focus on sexual orientation, saying,

> it is a rather amazing fact that, of the very many dimensions along which the genital activity of one person can be differentiated from that of another (dimensions that include preferences for certain acts, certain zones or sensations, certain physical types, a certain frequency, certain symbolic investments, certain relations of age or power, a certain species, a certain number of participants, and so on) precisely one, the gender of the object choice, emerged from the turn of the century, and has remained, as the dimension denoted by the now ubiquitous category of 'sexual orientation'.[40]

Think about it yourself. Can the important features of your sexuality be captured in a term relating to which gender you find attractive (bisexual, gay, straight, etc.) or would you need to describe other things – for example, if you were searching for somebody who might be sexually compatible on a dating website. You might want to consider, for example:

- The kinds of people you're attracted to in terms of other aspects such as physical appearance, age, personality, clothing, etc.

- The kinds of situations, images, roles, activities, or fantasies, if any, which excite you – and turn you off – physically and/or psychologically
- The kinds of physical sensations you enjoy and don't enjoy

Sexual configurations

Biological psychological research has recently begun to consider multiple dimensions of human sexuality rather than limiting itself to orientation on the basis of gender. In her framework for human sexuality, Sari Van Anders[41] reviews the biological and psychological research relating to the following dimensions:

- The physical sex of the person we're attracted to
- Their gender (how masculine, feminine, or androgynous they are, which may or may not match their physical sex) and
- The number of people we can be attracted to at the same time (whether we're monogamous or non-monogamous or something in between, see Chapter 4)

Van Anders also acknowledges there are probably many more possible dimensions, and we'll be considering a few of them over the coming chapters (particularly the level of sexual attraction we experience – from none to high, and where we are on spectrums of sexually submissive/dominant or passive/active).

So in order to measure sexuality completely we'd need something far more complex than a Kinsey scale or even a Klein grid. We'd need to imagine something like multiple Kinsey scales on these many different dimensions all intersecting and interweaving in complex ways. If that's not already complicated enough, sexual fluidity means where we're at on these multiple dimensions is probably shifting and changing over time. And – as Van Anders and Diamond point out – we may be in different places in terms of who we're sexually attracted to (if anyone), what we think about during solo sex (if anything), and who we have emotionally close or romantic relationships with (if anyone). We all have a unique *sexual configuration*, rather than a sexual orientation we share with a large proportion of the population.

Queer and intersectional sexualities

Sexual configurations theory is highly influenced by both queer and intersectional feminist theories.

While queer is often used simply as an umbrella term for sexualities and genders beyond the heterosexual and cisgender norms, queer theory and queer activism use it to mean anything that challenges or disrupts normative culture, particularly – but not exclusively – in relation to sexuality and gender.[42] So queer sexualities could look like:

- Any sexuality that challenged heteronormativity, including heterosexual people having non-normative kinds of sex (like threesomes or women penetrating male partners)
- Sexualities that trouble both heteronormativity and homonormativity[43] – the normative ways of embodying sexuality that have emerged in gay cultures
- Sexualities which go beyond binaries of attraction to men/women, such as bisexuality and pansexuality
- Sexualities unrelated to gender of attraction, given how linked that is to sexuality in hetero- and homonormativity, such as some asexual and kink sexualities (see Chapters 3 and 4)
- Sexualities that are open to changing over time, understanding queer as a verb (a doing word) rather than a noun (a fixed thing that we are)
- Sexualities that refuse and resist even the new normativities that emerge within queer communities of all kinds (e.g. hierarchies of queerness and concerns about being queer enough) and draw our attention to the oppressive systems and structures that can go, unchecked, within queer communities

This latter point brings us to the idea of intersectionality, from Black feminist Kimberlé Crenshaw: a perspective which is aligned with much Black feminist scholarship and activism which emphasises interconnection and interdependence as well as how oppression operates at the level of cultural systems and structures, communities, and relationships.[44]

Crenshaw's theory began with a legal case where Black women were being excluded from working at an automobile plant. The court found no evidence of discrimination because white women were being hired as administrative workers (no gender bias) and Black men were being hired for industrial jobs (no racial bias). Crenshaw argued we therefore need to see how axes of oppression like gender and race *intersect*.[45] Applying this to sexuality, we might consider a workplace where, following campaigns, white women experience less sexual harassment and Black men experience less racial harassment, but Black women still experience being objectified and receiving unwanted touch and comments on appearance and sexual interest because of the different ways misogyny and racism intersect in how Black women have been treated historically and currently.[46] For Black women who are also bisexual – another category which has historically been sexualised – this may restrict them from coming out or accessing LGBTQIA+ workplace support groups, for fear of facing even greater harassment if they do so.

Intersectional approaches draw our attention to how scientific projects of delineating certain sexualities as acceptable, good, or normal were interwoven with historical scientific projects of categorising certain race and class groups as superior or inferior (to justify colonialism and exploitation); attempting to prevent certain groups from reproducing, including 'lower class', immigrant, and disabled people; and creating or exaggerating gender differences in order to continue capitalist systems rooted in women working unpaid in the home to care for, and reproduce, the workforce.[47]

We can see the legacies of all these things in the continued operation of oppression in general and in relation to sexuality specifically. For example, ideals of sexual attractiveness remain overwhelmingly young, white, wealthy, abled, and slim (with anti-fatness itself being highly related to race-, class-, and gender-based oppression).[48] Many marginalised people experience being receiving abuse, unwanted attention, or lack of attention, on dating and hookup apps, due to pernicious stereotypes of certain racial groups being hypersexual, or non-sexual, or having certain kinds of bodies.[49] In sexual relationships, power differences between people on the basis of intersecting oppressions can have a significant impact on capacity to be in consent (see Chapter 4). So intersectional sexualities would be those where we're aware that the way our sexualities manifest is inextricably linked to how we're positioned on various axes of oppression. In Chapter 6 we'll explore more how colonialist and capitalist cultures show up in our sex lives.

NATURE, NURTURE, OR . . . SOMETHING ELSE?

Now we've explored how we understand sexuality, let's return to the other question about sexuality which has vexed psychologists (and other scientists) since the start: the question of what *causes* our sexuality.

If you remember back to the beginning of this chapter you'll remember that the questions of categorisation and causation were pretty much interlinked in early theories of sexuality. The first sexologists assumed that the sexual 'deviants' they classified were explainable by biological variation. Freud theorised that adult sexuality could be explained by people becoming fixated at one of the early stages of childhood sexual development and therefore not having developed to 'healthy' sexual maturity. In the last few decades the prevailing view has swung back to biology with the search for the 'gay gene' and for brain differences to account for sexual orientation.

These shifts demonstrate the way in which the question has often been put – in psychology and in wider culture – as 'nature or nurture?' Are gay people born that way or made that way? By now I hope you can already see there are problems with the way this question is framed. These mean any research attempting to answer it will be of limited value.

Problems with the question

First, framed in this way the question assumes there is normal sexual orientation (heterosexuality), and then there is sexual orientation which is different from that (homosexuality) and which requires explanation. Otherwise we'd be asking what caused heterosexuality too. As we've seen throughout this chapter, however, sexuality isn't binary. Even if we could pull out one dimension (gender of attraction) to focus on in this way, we'd need to account for the whole spectrum of possible attractions and their lack, rather than just attempting to explain one end of the spectrum.

Second, the question of causation often assumes there will be *one* explanation that accounts for all people who have a certain sexuality. Why are people gay? Why are people bi? These may sound like reasonable questions because we've heard them asked in this way so many times. As we'll see in later chapters the same tends to apply when psychologists search for explanations of other sexual identities and practices. Returning to what we learnt from Klein and Van Anders, we can see a problem with this. If – as seems to be the case – each of us has a unique sexual configuration where we sit in different places on a number of different dimensions, then it seems unlikely we could find universal explanations for sexuality. It's more likely that multiple elements are involved in shaping our sexuality, operating together in complex ways which differ from person to person. In addition to this, of course, we need explanations that can account for the shifts and changes many people experience over time – sexual fluidity – as well as the experiences of those whose sexuality seems to be more fixed.

Sedgwick, who we encountered earlier, has pointed out the nature/nurture binary is another binary that we need to question. Is it true that all aspects of human experience can be put down to either nature or nurture: either biological or social factors? She points out each time popular and scientific opinion has swung from nature to nurture or back again, it's always homosexuality that's seen as somehow deficient (for example, as being the result of overprotective mothers – nurture – or feminised brains – nature).

Psychologists Peter Hegarty and Felicia Pratto conducted a range of studies which illustrate this nicely. They found that psychologists, and people in general, when asked to explain a difference in sexual orientation or gender, tend to explain it in terms of how gay people differ from straight people or how women differ from men. For example, 'women did worse on that task because their brain activity is less focused than men' or 'gay men are more creative because they're more feminine than straight men'.[50] This is an example of *heteronormativity*.

The search for biological explanations of homosexuality is often justified by saying that if we can prove people are 'born gay' then gay people will be treated better. Hegarty and Pratto also found that people who believed this in biological explanations weren't any less homophobic than people who accepted more social explanations.[51]

The assumption that biological explanations will somehow legitimise homosexuality also reveals a common slippage people make when thinking about these issues. They often assume that something being biological makes it somehow more 'real' than something being social: if people are 'born gay' then they can't do anything about it, whereas if it was something that developed over time perhaps they could. There's confusion here between the question of nature vs. nurture and the question of something being determined vs. chosen. The two things don't map onto each other. Saying something is social, or learnt, is not the same as saying it's chosen (a lifestyle choice or a preference that could easily be otherwise). Take something that's clearly learnt socially – such as wearing clothes. The fact this is down to nurture rather than nature doesn't mean it would be easy to strip naked and walk down the street that way!

Biopsychosocial

All this discussion still risks accepting the premise that things can be divided into nature and nurture, biological and social, and this just isn't the case. As we saw when we explored sex and gender earlier, most aspects of human experiences are actually *biopsychosocial*:[52] a long word which means they involve our biology, our psychology, and the social world around us, with all of those things influencing each other in complex feedback loops, making it impossible to tease apart each element or the direction of any cause-effect relationships.

As neuroscientists such as Cordelia Fine have pointed out, the way we learn things is undeniably biopsychosocial. For example, if we live in a social world where kids are expected to ride a bike (social) we will likely start trying to do so and, as we learn (psychological), our neural connections will wire up in such a way that we remember how to do it and our body will start to habitually do what it needs to do to stay upright and move forward (biological). Obviously the connections work in the opposite direction too, in that our existing body and brain abilities and limitations (biological) will make learning to ride a bike more or less easy for us (psychological), which will influence how we experience the (social) world if it's easier or more difficult for us to join our friends on their bikes or to get from A to B. The processes of developing gender roles, or sexual attractions, are probably not so very different to this.

The diagram and table on the next page give you a (oversimplified) flavour of how some of these influences might work.

Biopsychosocial processes

Going around Figure 2.2 clockwise via the outer arrows and then counterclockwise via the inner arrows, I've provided some examples of how each operates, in relation to sexuality (Table 2.3).

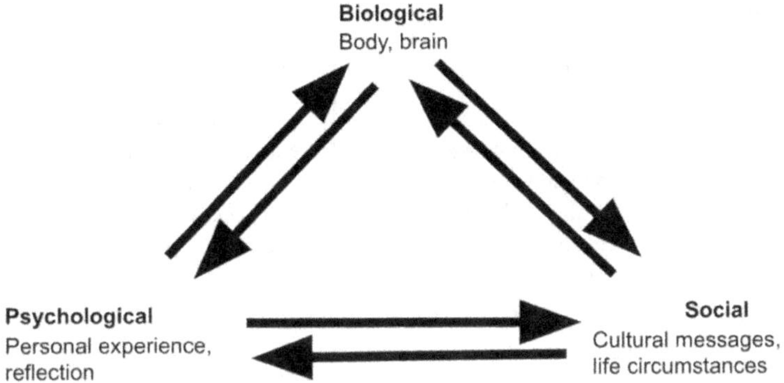

FIGURE 2.2 Biopsychosocial processes

TABLE 2.3 Biopsychosocial influences on each other

Direction of influence	*How it can operate*	*Examples*
Biological -> social	Our physiological characteristics mean we're treated in certain ways by the world around us	How much our body and brain functions conform to social norms of attractiveness in the time and place we live in
Social -> psychological	This impacts how we experience the world, and what opportunities are available to us	If we're regarded as attractive we'll have more potential partners and be treated better generally
Psychological -> biological	Our experiences shape our bodily habits and brain processes	If we're encouraged to be comfortable in our body we'll develop a more relaxed relationship with it – and with sex – than if we're not
Biological -> psychological	Hormonal levels and other features of our biology may point us in certain directions in terms of our desires and characteristics, opening up some experiential possibilities and closing down others	If we're born with the tendency to be more open to new experiences, or more wary, this may gradually develop – through our experiences – into more sexual openness or cautiousness in later life

(Continued)

TABLE 2.3 (Continued)

Direction of influence	*How it can operate*	*Examples*
Social -> biological	Cultural messages embed themselves on our bodies and brains. Social circumstances make certain sexual behaviours possible or impossible	We learn to move in certain ways, or think in certain ways, because of the social expectations, about a person of our gender, race and class, for example If we spend all our time in an entirely same-sex environment like some prisons and military environments this will influence what sexual opportunities are physically available to us which may shape our sexual behaviours and attractions
Psychological -> social	We can resist cultural messages and social norms through our actions, potentially opening up different cultural possibilities	Perhaps we get involved in campaigns for sexual rights or sex education which influence the messages people who come after us receive about sex and sexuality

It might be helpful to pick one aspect of your own sexuality and work through the diagram considering how the different aspects might be interlinked for you. Again, it's important to emphasise here that something having psychological and/or social elements does not make it any less 'real', 'legitimate', or 'fixed' than it being purely biological – if it's even possible to draw such distinctions given the way our experiences and cultural world write themselves onto our bodies and brains.

As we move through the rest of this book it's particularly important to remember that the way our culture views sexuality will influence how available different sexual identities or practices are to us: for example, if we live in a time and place where homosexuality is viewed as a sin, a crime, a sickness, or an acceptable identity. Cultural shifts in how women having sex with women are viewed may partially explain increases in the number of women having same-sex experiences in recent years.[53] And remember the differences the YouGov survey found between people of various generations reporting same-sex attraction (a quarter of all adults, but half of young adults).

CONCLUSIONS

Going back to our summary of assumptions that have often been made in psychology – and in wider culture – about sexuality, let's rethink the list from the start of this chapter:

- Sexuality isn't *binary* (many people are not purely homo- or heterosexual).
- So we can't *categorise* people into one of two boxes on the basis of sexual 'orientation' – it's more like a spectrum.
- Except actually it's more like multiple spectrums because there are so many different dimensions to sexuality (beyond what sex/gender we're attracted to – and, by the way, that isn't binary either) – therefore we each have a unique *sexual configuration*.
- Sexuality is *fluid* – people experience some aspects of their sexuality as dynamic and changing over time as well as some as more stable.
- Sexuality is *biopsychosocial*: all of these elements combine in complex ways to shape our unique dynamic sexual configuration.

All this clearly has major implications for the questions we ask in psychology about sexuality, and how we go about answering them. It also has wider implications for how we teach kids about sexuality or how we campaign for sexual and gender equality. Perhaps we need to move away from the 'majority norm – minority other' models towards a model of sexual and gender diversity. Over the next few chapters you'll see how such a model might be a better fit for other aspects of sex too, such as our levels of sexual desire, the sexual practices we enjoy, and the kinds of sexual relationships we engage in.

NOTES

1 Epstein, D., O'Flynn, S., & Telford, D. (2003). *Silenced sexualities in schools and universities*. Trentham Books; Winter, J. (2022). What should a queer children's book do. *The New Yorker*. Available from: newyorker.com/news/annals-of-education/lgbt-books-kids-ban

2 Collier, K. L., Bos, H. M., & Sandfort, T. G. (2013). Homophobic name-calling among secondary school students and its implications for mental health. *Journal of Youth and Adolescence*, 42 (3), 363–375.

3 Although there are many recent, more inclusive, versions of psychoanalysis, which we'll touch on in Chapter 6.

4 Barker, M. (2007). Heteronormativity and the exclusion of bisexuality in psychology. In V. Clarke & E. Peel (Eds.), *Out in psychology: Lesbian, gay, bisexual, trans, and queer perspectives* (pp. 86–118). Wiley.

5 See also Stelzl, M., & Stairs, B. (2014). The construction of sexuality knowledge in human sexuality textbooks. In Anna Pilińska and Harmony Siganporia (Eds.), *All equally real: Femininities and masculinities today*(pp. 279–293). Brill.

6 Carey, B. (2005). Straight, gay or lying: Bisexuality revisited. *New York Times*, 5.

7 Rieger, G., Chivers, M. L., & Bailey, J. M. (2005). Sexual arousal patterns of bisexual men. *Psychological Science*, *16* (8), 579–584.

8 Rosenthal, A. M., Sylva, D., Safron, A., & Bailey, J. M. (2011). Sexual arousal patterns of bisexual men revisited. *Biological Psychology*, 88 (1), 112–115.

9 See Feinstein, B. A., & Galupo, M. P. (2020). Bisexual orientation cannot be reduced to arousal patterns. *Proceedings of the National Academy of Sciences*, *117* (50), 31575–31576.

10 Barker, M. J., & Iantaffi, A. (2019). *Life isn't binary*. Jessica Kingsley.

11 See Shaw, J. (2022). *Bi: The hidden culture, history and science of bisexuality*. Canongate books; Shearing, L. & Mehta, V. (2024). *It ain't over till the bisexual speaks*. Jessica Kingsley.

12 See ons.gov.uk/census/censustransformationprogramme/questiondevelopment/sexualorientationquestiondevelopmentforcensus2021

13 Kinsey, A. C., Pomeroy, W. B., & Martin, C. E. (1948). *Sexual behavior in the human male*. Indiana University Press; Kinsey, A. C., Pomeroy, W. B., &

Martin, C. E. (1953). *Sexual behavior in the human female*. Indiana University Press.

14 The film *Kinsey* is a great starting place if you're interested in finding out more about Kinsey's life and work. For details on the research findings see https://www.kinseyinstitute.org/research/index.php

15 Lesbian, Gay, Bisexual, Transgender, Queer+. ougov.co.uk/international/articles/37846-international-survey-how-supportive-would-britons-

16 yougov.co.uk/society/articles/23882-one-five-young-people-identify-gay-lesbian-or-bise, yougov.co.uk/topics/society/trackers/how-brits-describe-their-sexuality

17 For example, check out the different figures across time and culture on the Wikipedia page about sexual orientation: http://en.wikipedia.org/wiki/Demographics_of_sexual_orientation

18 Klein, F., Sepekoff, B., & Wolf, T. J. (1985). Sexual orientation: A multi-variable dynamic process. *Journal of Homosexuality, 11* (1–2), 35–49.

19 Klein, F. (2014). *The bisexual option*. Routledge.

20 Diamond, L. M. (2009). *Sexual fluidity*. Harvard University Press.

21 Chivers, M. L., Seto, M. C., & Blanchard, R. (2007). Gender and sexual orientation differences in sexual response to sexual activities versus gender of actors in sexual films. *Journal of Personality and Social Psychology, 93* (6), 1108.

22 Savin-Williams, R. C., Joyner, K., & Rieger, G. (2012). Prevalence and stability of self-reported sexual orientation identity during young adulthood. *Archives of Sexual Behavior, 41* (1), 103–110.

23 Mock, S. E., & Eibach, R. P. (2012). Stability and change in sexual orientation identity over a 10-year period in adulthood. *Archives of Sexual Behavior, 41* (3), 641–648.

24 Loviscky, A. J., Vescio, T. K., Yamaguchi-Pedroza, K., Sullivan, J. T., & Basar, D. (2024). Hegemonic masculinity and sexism. In Todd D. Nelson (Ed.), *Handbook of prejudice, stereotyping, and discrimination* (pp. 205–250). Routledge.

25 Pathela, P., Hajat, A., Schillinger, J., Blank, S., Sell, R., & Mostashari, F. (2006). Discordance between sexual behavior and self-reported sexual identity: A population-based survey of New York City men. *Annals of Internal Medicine, 145* (6), 416–425.

26 For an overview of research on sexual fluidity, see Katz-Wise, S. L., & Todd, K. P. (2022). The current state of sexual fluidity research. *Current Opinion in Psychology*, 48, 101497.

27 Jowett, A., Brady, G., Goodman, S., Pillinger, C., & Bradley, L. (2020). *Conversion therapy: An evidence assessment and qualitative study*. Research Report. Government Equalities Office, UK Government. Available from: e-space.mmu.ac.uk/633306/1/2020_12_15_Conversion_Therapy_Reserach_Report_AJ_edited_clean_4_.pdf

28 Fausto-Sterling, A. (2000). *Sexing the body: Gender politics and the construction of sexuality*. Basic Books, p. 31. For a simple overview of these ideas see Fausto-Sterling, A. (2012). *Sex/gender: Biology in a social world*. Routledge. See also Fausto-Sterling, A. (2018). Why sex is not binary. *The New York Times*, 25.

29 Joel, D., & Vikhanski, L. (2019). *Gender mosaic: Beyond the myth of the male and female brain*. Hachette UK.

30 Fine, C. (2010). *Delusions of gender*. Icon Books.

31 Herdt, G. H. (1993). *Third sex, third gender: Beyond sexual dimorphism in culture and history*. Zone Books.

32 ons.gov.uk/news/news/firstcensusestimatesongenderidentityandsexualorientation; Titman, N. (2014). *How many people in the United Kingdom are nonbinary?* Available from: practicalandrogyny.com/2014/12/16/how-many-people-in-the-uk-are-nonbinary/

33 Joel, D., Tarrasch, R., Berman, Z., Mukamel, M., & Ziv, E. (2014). Queering gender: Studying gender identity in 'normative' individuals. *Psychology & Sexuality*, 5 (4), 291–321.

34 For more on this, see: Barker, M. J., & Scheele, J. (2019). *Gender: A graphic guide*. Icon Books; Iantaffi, A., & Barker, M. J. (2017). *How to understand your gender*. Jessica Kingsley; Iantaffi, A., & Barker, M. J. (2019). *Life isn't binary*. Jessica Kingsley.

35 Bem, S. L. (1981). Gender schema theory: A cognitive account of sex typing. *Psychological Review*, 88 (4), 354. Bem, S. L. (1995). Dismantling gender polarization and compulsory heterosexuality: Should we turn the volume down or up? *Journal of Sex Research*, 32 (4), 329–334.

36 Hayfield, N. (2020). *Bisexual and pansexual identities: Exploring and challenging invisibility and invalidation*. Routledge.

37 Jeffs, L., & Oakley, S. (2025). *Do ask, do tell: Queer life, love and culture laid bare*. Pan Macmillan; Guyan, K. (2022). *Queer data*. Bloomsbury; rewriting-the-rules.com/sex/sapiosexuality.

38 Bowes-Catton, H., Barker, M., & Richards, C. (2011). 'I didn't know that I could feel this relaxed in my body': Using visual methods to research bisexual people's embodied experiences of identity and space. In P. Reavey (Ed.), *Visual methods in psychology: Using and interpreting images in qualitative research* (pp. 255–270). Routledge.

39 Turley, E. L., King, N., & Monro, S. (2018). 'You want to be swept up in it all': Illuminating the erotic in BDSM. *Psychology & Sexuality*, 9 (2), 148–160.

40 Sedgwick, E. K. (1990). *Epistemology of the closet*. Prentice Hall, p. 8.

41 van Anders, S. M. (2015). Beyond sexual orientation: Integrating gender/sex and diverse sexualities via sexual configurations theory. *Archives of Sexual Behavior*, 1–3744(5), 1177–1213; queensu.ca/psychology/van-anders-lab/assets/docs/SCTzine.pwe aredf

42 Barker, M. J. (2016). *Queer: A graphic history*. Icon Books.

43 Robinson, B. A. (2016). Heteronormativity and homonormativity. In N. Naples (Ed.), *The Wiley Blackwell encyclopedia of gender and sexuality studies* (pp. 1–3). Wiley Blackwell.

44 Collins, P. H., & Bilge, S. (2020). *Intersectionality*. John Wiley & Sons; Hooks, B. (2000). *Feminist theory: From margin to center*. Pluto Press.

45 Crenshaw, K. (2015). Why intersectionality can't wait. *The Washington Post*, 24.09.

46 Noble, D., & Palmer, L. A. (2022). Misogynoir: Anti-blackness, patriarchy, and refusing the wrongness of black women. In Shirley Anne Tate and Encarnación Gutiérrez Rodríguez (Eds.), *The Palgrave handbook of critical race and gender* (pp. 227–245). Springer International Publishing.

47 See Barker, M-J. (2017). *BACP good practice in action fact sheet 095: Gender, Sexual, and Relationship Diversity (GSRD)*. British Association of Counselling & Psychotherapy. Available from: rewriting-the-rules.com/gender-sexual-diversity-lgbt-mental-health-resources

48 Da'Shaun, L. H. (2021). *Belly of the beast: The politics of anti-fatness as anti-blackness*. North Atlantic Books.

49 Hakim, J., Cummings, J., & Young, I., (2025). *Digital intimacies: Queer men and smartphones in times of crisis*. Bloomsbury.

50 Hegarty, P., & Pratto, F. (2004). The differences that norms make: Empiricism, social constructionism, and the interpretation of group differences. *Sex Roles*, 50 (7–8), 445–453.

51 Hegarty, P., & Pratto, F. (2001). Sexual orientation beliefs: Their relationship to anti-gay attitudes and biological determinist arguments. *Journal of Homosexuality*, 41 (1), 121–135.

52 Denman, C. (2017). *Sexuality: A biopsychosocial approach*. Palgrave Macmillan.

53 NATSAL (2013). *Sexual attitudes and lifestyles in Britain: Highlights from Natsal-3*. Available from: www.natsal.ac.uk/media/2102/natsal-infographic.pdf. Natsal-4 was conducted between 2022 and 2024, but the findings were not available at the time of writing.

3

'PROPER' SEX

As you saw in the last chapter, the psychology of sex has generally focused on sex in the context of sexuality or 'sexual orientation'. This is the sex-related topic often given the most room in psychology textbooks and psychology journals. However, when you considered the question 'What is sex?' in the introduction to this book, sexuality probably wasn't the first thing which sprang to mind. What we tend to mean by sex is 'the sex act', 'having sex', or 'sexual intercourse'.

The areas of psychology that have devoted most attention to this topic are the ones which border on counselling, psychotherapy, and psychiatry: areas such as counselling psychology and clinical psychology where psychologists work therapeutically with clients or patients to ease their suffering. So that's what we'll concentrate on in this chapter, with a particular focus on sex therapy or psychosexual therapy – the kind of therapy that focuses on sexual problems.

Psychology, psychiatry, and psychotherapy have historically categorised sexual problems (or 'disorders') in two main ways: the sexual *dysfunctions* and the *paraphilias*. Sexual dysfunctions are difficulties that get in the way of a person having what's regarded as *functional* sex. Paraphilias are *abnormal* sexual desires. In this chapter we'll focus on functional versus dysfunctional sex to explore what's regarded as

DOI: 10.4324/9781003728979-3

the 'proper' sex people should be having. In the next chapter we'll turn our attention to the normal versus abnormal sex distinction. As always we'll attend to the ways psychology and related disciplines have been involved in *constructing* these functional/dysfunctional and normal/abnormal distinctions as well as to what psychological theories and research in this area can tell us about sex.

WHAT IS SEX?

It's useful to start by asking ourselves this question again. Think about it for yourself: if somebody tells you they've had sex, or they want to have sex, what do you think they mean?

I feel like I have a fair sense of our wider cultural understanding of sex because I once spent a long time analysing sex manuals and other forms of sex advice for a piece of psychological research.[1] In all I read sixty-five sex advice books – not something I'd necessarily recommend! I also looked at a large number of newspaper problem pages and websites. My colleagues on the project studied sex-related TV documentaries and magazine articles. So between us we got a pretty good sense of how sex advice media understands sex.

We found that what sex advice generally means by sex is penis-in-vagina (PIV) intercourse with the goal of orgasm. On average around 17% of the content of the books I looked at were dedicated to PIV intercourse, compared to 5% on oral sex, 4% on manual sex (using hands), 3% on various forms of kinky sex, 2% on solo sex (or masturbation), and 1% on anal sex. The position of these topics in the books was also telling. By and large things like oral sex, manual sex, and solo sex were covered earlier in the books in sections on 'foreplay', suggesting they don't count as 'proper sex' in themselves, just as precursors to the 'real thing'. The books covered solo sex almost exclusively as a way of getting better at 'proper sex' by figuring out how you like to be touched or learning how to last longer, for example. Topics such as anal sex, kinky sex, and sex toys were covered later in the books in sections on 'spicing up your sex life'. So again they weren't part of the 'main course' part of the book, but rather additional 'side orders' which only some people might want to try.

The point of most of the sex advice books was to help readers to sustain a good sex life throughout a long-term relationship – something we'll come back to later in the chapter. Again you can see what they meant by sex in the guidance they gave for how to do this. The bulk of the advice focused on varying the positions of PIV sex. Indeed some of the books consisted almost entirely of photographs or diagrams of different bodily arrangements through which you could have PIV sex. Some books also suggested having PIV sex in different locations, or wearing different clothes, or sometimes adding sex toys or other kinds of sex into PIV sex in order to maximise the chance of both people reaching orgasm. However, PIV intercourse was almost always central.

'So what?' you might be thinking, 'of course sex means PIV intercourse, and of course the point of sex is to get an orgasm'. As with the cultural assumptions about sexuality we covered in the previous chapter, these things often *seem* obvious because they've come to be so widely taken for granted. Once we start to unpack them, however, we can see how they came to be this way because of the particular historical journey that has brought us to this point. Then we can turn to other theories and research to see some problems with the prevailing view, as well as how we might usefully take a different approach.

PENISES, VAGINAS, AND ORGASMS

So how did we get to this point: PIV leading to orgasm as the 'gold standard' form of sex which we're all meant to be striving for?

Back to Freud

Again we need to go back to Freud, whose theories of sex – whether we know it or not – have had a marked impact on how we understand sex today.

Before Freud, the early sexologists with their biological focus generally drew on Darwinian thinking and therefore saw the whole purpose of sex as procreation. This explains their desire to categorise and explain any sexual practices and desires that *couldn't* lead to reproduction. What Freud proposed – which was so radical at the time – was the idea the purpose of sex was *pleasure*, not procreation. He noticed the bulk of the sex which people had – and wanted – didn't have the goal of reproduction. In fact, where procreation is a risk, people often go to great lengths to avoid pregnancy.

Freud's theories didn't completely eradicate the view that 'normal, natural' sex should be that which *could* lead to procreation. You've probably heard this idea expressed yourself – it still haunts many discussions about sexuality. However, his ideas certainly opened up other possibilities. You'll see in the next chapter how research has found both humans and other animals have sex for many reasons other than reproducing.

Historians and sociologists of sex suggest Freud's thinking about pleasure – along with societal changes happening at the time – meant sex became viewed as something like a leisure pursuit: an important element of the married lives of the middle classes. This notion filtered out to society more widely. Then improvements in contraception, particularly the 'sexual revolution' of the pill, took us towards the current view – as expressed in the sex advice books – that sexual satisfaction is a key element of a 'successful relationship'.

The aim of sex

Thinking back to the previous chapter you might remember that Freud proposed healthy, mature sexuality involved a certain sexual *object* (the 'opposite sex') and a certain sexual *aim*. It's this aim that developed the notion of PIV sex as the gold standard. Basically Freud proposed that all children go through several stages of psychosexual development, theorising that at each stage, the child's libido focuses on a different *erogenous zone* or bodily source of pleasure (Table 3.1).[2]

TABLE 3.1 Freud's stages of psychosexual development

Age	*Stage*	*Normal development*
0–1	Oral	Children are preoccupied with their mouths because they feed from the breast. They explore the world orally.
1–3	Anal	Children fixate on their anus. As they become able to control their bowels and bladder, they learn the value of self-control and delayed gratification.
3–6	Phallic	Children become interested in their genitals and begin to masturbate. They notice differences between people's genitals. Unconsciously, they want to possess their opposite-sex parent and are jealous of their same-sex parent (Oedipus complex, see Chapter 2). The conflict is resolved when they learn to identify with their same-sex parent instead of regarding them as a rival.
6-puberty	Latency	Having successfully repressed their libidos, children now go through a period of latency, and they don't experience sexual desire.
Puberty onwards	Genital	Sexual desire re-emerges, focused on the genitals. Women now reach orgasm vaginally instead of clitorally. Sexual activity is partnered rather than solo.

From this table you can see how Freud's theories present PIV sex as the proper, mature form of sexual activity with orgasm as the goal. You can also see how solo sex and oral, anal, and manual sex are seen as less mature or healthy forms of sex. Like same-sex attraction, lack of sexual desire is regarded as an immature childhood 'phase'. Finally – and importantly – you can see how sexuality became linked to our personalities and identities beyond sex. Freud proposed that some people become *fixated* at earlier stages of psychosexual development, which results in them being a certain kind of person: anally retentive people being obsessive and perfectionist, orally fixated people being naive and immature, and so on.

Even if many psychologists today are sceptical of these ideas of early childhood sexuality and the operations of unconscious processes, they've clearly left their mark on our assumptions about what 'proper sex' should be like and the place it should have in people's lives.

Masters of sex

The other people who had perhaps the most marked impact on our current understandings of 'proper sex' are William Masters and Virginia Johnson. You might have seen the TV series *Masters of Sex*, based on their lives and work.

William Masters was a gynaecologist and Virginia Johnson was his assistant who later became his partner. Like Alfred Kinsey, who we met in the previous chapter, their focus was on the biological and physiological aspects of sex. Unlike Kinsey – and perhaps partly because of the huge controversy surrounding Kinsey's research – Masters and Johnson weren't driven to study the diversity of human sexual behaviour. Rather, they focused on discovering how 'normal' sex worked. Later, they turned their focus on how to help people whose sexual experiences didn't follow this pattern to conform to it.

Masters and Johnson also wanted to study the physiology and anatomy of sex directly, rather than just hearing people's *reports* of what they did sexually. For this reason they observed hundreds of people taking part in over 10,000 'cycles of sexual response' under laboratory conditions, while taking measurements of heart rate, blood pressure, etc. They observed PIV sex, masturbation, and 'artificial coition' (masturbation using a dildo-like device which simulated PIV sex while filming it 'from the inside').

The sexual response cycle

The major outcome of Masters and Johnson's research was their four-stage model of sexual response:[3]

1. Excitement: Erectile tissues such as the penis and clitoris become engorged.
2. Plateau: The clitoris or testes retract as orgasm approaches.
3. Orgasm: There are a series of rhythmical muscular contractions in the vagina and uterus, or penis and urethra. Pulse rate and blood pressure peak, and facial grimacing often occurs.
4. Resolution: Breathing returns to normal and signs of arousal gradually subside. For men this is followed by a refractory period of minutes or hours before arousal can happen again, whereas women do not have such a period and can experience multiple orgasms.

So from Masters and Johnson we get the idea that there's a *sexual response cycle*: a kind of script, or set of stages, which sex should follow. This includes ideas about how our bodies should respond at each stage, and the 'normal' length of time each stage should take. You might want to reflect on this yourself: does it match your own experiences of sex if you've had sex? If you were going to divide sex into stages, which ones would you choose? You'll see in a moment that people have had different ideas about this.

Masters and Johnson did dispel some of the myths which were circulating about sex at the time they were writing, and, like Kinsey and his team, their work helpfully got people talking somewhat more openly about sex. For example, they challenged the 'bigger=better' assumption, finding penis size made very little difference to women's experiences of PIV sex because vaginas are elastic and accommodate themselves to the size of a penis. Also, the size of a flaccid penis isn't a good guide to how large it will be when it's erect because they expand by different amounts.

Importantly, Masters and Johnson also demonstrated there was no physiological difference between 'vaginal' and 'clitoral' orgasms. If you remember, Freud saw 'vaginal' orgasms as more mature. However, given the clitoris is actually a large organ which extends back internally through the body, the sensations of orgasm are always produced by the same network of nerves, whether they're stimulated internally or externally or both. Although Masters and Johnson found no difference between these types of orgasm, they didn't manage to let go of the assumption that women *should* be able to orgasm through PIV sex alone and that being unable to do so was a form of dysfunction.

Shaping the current view of sex

From this quick tour through how understandings of sex have shifted over the last hundred years or so, you can again see the role of theories and research in this area in both *informing* us about sex and in simultaneously *constructing* certain understandings which influence how people think about – and experience – themselves sexually. For example, a woman who orgasmed only through manual stimulation might – in the late nineteenth century – have seen herself as a sexual deviant (if she could even read the early sexological texts, some of which were written in Latin deliberately so as not to be accessible to uneducated people). In the early twentieth century she might, through psychoanalysis, have come to understand herself as sexually immature and fixated. And in the 1960s she might have been encouraged by Masters and Johnsons' findings but still have sought a way to orgasm from PIV sex – perhaps through the burgeoning field of psychosexual therapy.

Similarly, just think what a radical change solo sex has gone through: from the point over a century ago where there were devices to prevent people from masturbating and it was thought to cause all kinds of physical and psychological problems, to the point now where it's actually prescribed by sex therapists to help people with sexual problems – although masturbating to online pornography has perhaps replaced masturbation in general as the cultural bogeyman (see Chapter 5).

These changes over time demonstrate that our psychological and other scientific knowledge is, at least in part, rooted in the prevailing cultural norms – as well as contributing to them. This means that it could be otherwise, which is an important thought to take forward as we consider how we understand sex psychologically today.

FUNCTIONAL AND DYSFUNCTIONAL SEX?

Masters and Johnson's sexual response cycle was revised slightly by sex therapist Helen Singer Kaplan in the 1970s because it didn't include the feeling of sexual desire people often experience before they actually become physiologically excited or aroused.[4] Kaplan's cycle included just three stages: desire, arousal, and orgasm. This has become the blueprint for psychiatric, psychological, and psychotherapeutic categories of sexual *dysfunctions*, or *disorders*, since then, most of which involve a person struggling with one of these stages.

The bible for psychiatrists and other kinds of mental health professionals is the American Psychiatric Association's Diagnostic and Statistical Manual (DSM).[5] This weighty tome lists and describes all of the common 'mental disorders' so that medics and other practitioners can all diagnose people according to the same sets of criteria: the boxes you have to tick in order to be classified as depressed, anxious, or having a phobia, for example. Outside the US, some bodies also use the World Health Organization's International Statistical Classification of Diseases (ICD), which provides similar lists and generally follows the DSM, with very similar categories and criteria, at least in the area of sex and sexuality. Both the DSM and the ICD include sections on sexual dysfunctions and sections on paraphilias (which we'll come to in the next chapter).

The sexual dysfunctions

The DSM has been revised every decade or so since the first version in the 1950s and was on its fifth edition at the time of writing (DSM-5-TR). The sexual dysfunctions it lists are based around

Kaplan's revision of Masters and Johnson's sexual response cycle. Thus, there are categories relating to lack of desire or sexual interest (*desire*); lack of arousal and 'erectile disorder' (*arousal*); and 'female orgasmic disorder' and 'delayed ejaculation' (*orgasm*). In addition to these there are categories of 'premature (early) ejaculation' and of 'penetration disorder' (struggling to be penetrated due to tension or pain). You might want to think for a moment whether you've ever experienced any of these things yourself. If so, you'll see later that you share this with at least half of the population.

Looking at these categories gives us a clear idea of what the authors of the DSM consider to be 'functional' as well as 'dysfunctional' sex. Clearly people must go through the full sexual response cycle for functional sex to have occurred. They need to experience sexual *desire*, they need to become *aroused*, and they need to reach *orgasm*. Also PIV sex is obviously an essential feature, given it's considered to be a disorder if a vagina is not able to be penetrated, if a penis can't become erect enough to penetrate, and if ejaculation happens 'prematurely', in other words before penetration has happened.

There's also a tendency, these days, to see sexual 'dysfunctions' as primarily physiological problems which require a medical fix. Masters and Johnson assumed around 90% of sexual problems had a psychological origin and only 10% an organic one, whereas more recent claims have almost reversed this to 80% organic and 20% psychological.[6] We can see this in the massive popular interest in Viagra and other treatments for erectile dysfunction, as well as the race to find the Holy Grail of a female Viagra which would enhance women's libido.[7] It's intriguing to see the focus has been on getting men to have erections and getting women to want sex. This reveals some of our wider cultural assumptions about gender and sex.

In addition to medical treatments, sex therapists teach clients various physical techniques to address their sexual dysfunctions. These include stopping stimulation at various points for people with premature ejaculation; inserting a series of increasingly large dilators for people whose vaginas are too tense for PIV sex; and sensate focus, where couples who have sexual problems build up gradually from non-genital touching, to genital touching and eventually PIV.

So what's the problem with this model of sexual function and dysfunction? One useful question to ask yourself about any way of understanding things you come across in psychology is 'who does it exclude and who does it include?' and then to consider the implications for both groups of people. You might want to reflect on that question for a moment before reading on.

Exclusions

In terms of who it excludes, the functional/dysfunctional model of sex we've been looking at definitely assumes that people should have sexual desire, get aroused, and reach orgasm. As we'll see in the next section, although there have been some positive moves in this area, this excludes many asexual people who don't experience sexual attraction.

The model also clearly sees functional sex as sex which involves a penis penetrating a vagina. This excludes all people whose main sexual activities don't involve this, for example, those who prefer solo sex or kinky sex (which we'll look at in the next chapter) as well as couples whose combined sets of genitals are two penises or two vulvas. If the kinds of sex which are common in same-sex relationships were seen as just as proper or functional as PIV sex, then, along with penetration disorder, we should see categories of sexual dysfunction relating to being unable to control your gag reflex, having a tense anal sphincter, and perhaps repetitive strain injury. There should also be a category for women who orgasm or ejaculate prematurely. Some women do experience problems in orgasming too very quickly, but of course this does not interfere with PIV sex so there's no diagnostic category for it.[8]

The risk here is that although the DSM and sex therapists don't explicitly say that LGB people aren't having proper sex, this is what's implied by the fact the categories and treatments relate overwhelmingly to a certain form of heteronormative sex.

Inclusions

The implication that PIV sex is the right, best, or only proper kind of sex is also bad for people who *are* included in this model of sex. Even if you *can* have PIV sex, that doesn't mean it's the kind of sex you'll enjoy most. Also it involves far more risk of pregnancy and Sexually Transmitted Infections (STIs) than many other forms of sex. So it might be helpful if our model of sex included all forms of sex as equally valid and helped people to experience other kinds of sex in addition to PIV sex.

Feminist psychologists have pointed out some serious gender issues with the functional/dysfunctional model. First, the category of delayed ejaculation for men supports the common assumption that sex is over when the man ejaculates. While women's orgasms are regarded as important, they aren't generally seen as the *essential* component of sex male ejaculation is, by either sex advice or by sex therapy. You can see how this filters into the everyday experience of the 'orgasm gap'.[9]

We can also see this prioritising of men's sexual experience in the focus on vaginas rather than clitorises in the DSM. The clitoris is the part of the body which is equivalent to the penis and which enables arousal and orgasm. So why do the categories of sexual dysfunction, and measures of arousal such as the vaginal photoplethysmograph that we covered in the last chapter, focus so much on vaginas? Women don't need their vaginas to be penetrated in order to have sexual pleasure, and there are also many other forms of sexual pleasure available to men beyond penetrating a vagina. In fact, research on women's sexuality has found that the majority (around 70%) of them can't orgasm from PIV alone:[10] they need some kind of external stimulation of their clitoris in addition to – or instead of – vaginal stimulation. So why do we focus so much on PIV sex?

Sex manuals often search desperately for the one sexual position which would stimulate the external clitoris at the same time as allowing PIV: this is often called the CAT or coital alignment technique. However, in all the mainstream sex advice books I looked at, I never saw the sexual position where a woman lies on top of a man and takes his penis between her legs to rub her clitoris against. This is at least as likely as CAT to be pleasurable for both parties, but of course it doesn't include PIV so it's not considered.

Even the everyday language we have around sex demonstrates the focus on PIV, with men as the active people in sex and women as passive recipients. We talk of 'penetrative' sex, when 'enveloping' sex would be equally valid, and use euphemisms like 'nail' and 'screw'. The multimillion-selling classic self-help book *Mars and Venus in the Bedroom* explicitly states women should sometimes lay there 'like a block of wood', and that sex is a natural male need in a way it isn't for women.[11]

This gendered view of sex is bad for everyone. Obviously it excludes anybody whose gender and/or body doesn't fit the simple male/female binary – as we discussed in the last chapter. It also prevents us from seeing the similarities between, and the variations within, each gender category. For example, there are many similarities in the ways our genitals work – because they all began the same physiologically when we were in the womb. There's also a lot of variety between different people of the same gender about how active or passive they like being sexually, what kind of stimulation they enjoy, and so on.

The 'active initiating man, passive receiving woman' model which we currently have often disempowers women – to the point many have very little idea what actually turns them on because they're so focused on another person's pleasure rather than their own. The model also pressures men to act as unemotional machines, ever ready for sex, and focused purely on their 'performance'.[12] The idea that soft penises are 'dysfunctional' reinforces these kinds of stereotypes, leading to feelings of failure in men who don't 'measure up', and fear of failure in those who do. It also exacerbates the general cultural pressure on men not to be soft and gentle or open about their emotions.[13]

All of these expectations make communicating openly about sex very difficult due to the shame and stigma attached to admitting the PIV active man/passive woman model of sex doesn't work so well for us. We'll return to what sex therapy might look like if it took a wider perspective on what counted as sex towards the end of the chapter. Meanwhile, let's focus a bit more closely on a few of the other underlying assumptions about sex in the current model.

A BASIC HUMAN DRIVE?

One common idea about sex which underlies the model we've been exploring is that sex is necessary or *imperative*. Most sex advice books put forward the view that it's healthy to be sexual or even that sex is a natural human need akin to eating or breathing. They also claim sex is vital for relationships: it's the glue that holds a relationship together, and having less – or no – sex will inevitably lead to the end of a relationship. Think whether you've heard these ideas yourself and where. Do you agree or disagree that sex is an essential part of being human and necessary in order for relationships to work?

Historically we can see where these ideas of sex as essential for individuals and for relationships came from. Remember earlier in the chapter when we saw that Freud's theories linked our sexual aim to being a certain kind of person? Our sexual preferences became an inherent feature of our identity according to this model. Also we saw how sex historically became regarded as part of having a successful marriage.

Obviously this *sexual imperative* is useful for selling people books which advise people on how to keep having sex, but is there any validity to it apart from that? Or might it be damaging?

Asexuality

One group of people who've helped to challenge these commonly held assumptions in recent years has been *asexual* – or ace – communities. Asexual people are people who don't experience sexual attraction.

Thanks to online spaces like the Asexuality Visibility and Education Network (AVEN) it's become easier for asexual people to build communities and for ace experiences to be researched and communicated about, more widely.[14]

In the past psychologists and psychiatrists assumed 'lack of sexual attraction' was a sexual dysfunction, and asexual people would have been diagnosed with 'hypoactive sexual desire disorder' or similar. However, psychologist Lori Brotto's work in this area[15] meant the DSM-5 made it clear that asexual people should not be diagnosed in this way – or treated for any disorder. Research has demonstrated people don't experience any distress or relationship difficulties due to being asexual: the only difficulty is the stigma they receive from other people who don't understand asexuality. For example, studies with asexual people have found many had been treated in hostile ways by others, often being told their sexuality was just a phase, that they hadn't met the right person yet, being given sex toys, or even being sexual assaulted by people who said they wanted to 'cure' their asexuality.[16]

Asexuality helps us to see that many aspects of sexual experience are on a continuum, as we saw in the previous chapter in gender of attraction. One of these aspects is the amount of sexual attraction and/or desire we experience. The common view is that we *should* all conform to some normative amount of sexual desire, having sex a similar 'average' number of times per week. Understanding desire as a continuum, we can acknowledge some people will experience high levels of sexual feelings, some low, and some none at all. It can be as healthy not to experience sexual desire as to have a libido in any range.

Research on the diversity of asexual experiences is useful for opening our understanding of the different ways sexual attraction, desire, and arousal can work. Some asexual people are celibate (don't have sex) and some celibate people are asexual. However, just as there are celibate people who do have sexual desires but choose not to act on them, there are also asexual people who choose to have sex sometimes, even though they don't personally feel desire, for example, in order to give a partner sexual pleasure. Some asexual people are completely averse to sex, some feel more neutral about it. Some *grey-A* and *demisexual* people occasionally experience sexual attraction and see themselves as somewhere on the spectrum from asexual to sexual. For example, they might feel sexual but only with one specific person or enjoy solo sex but not sex with others. As with gender of attraction, some people experience their asexuality as fluid and changeable over time, others as fixed. Many asexual people want romantic or partner relationships, whereas *aromantic* (aro) asexual people do not.[17] We'll return to what we might all learn from ace and aro communities in Chapter 6.

The sexual imperative reconsidered

We can see from asexual experiences that sex is *not* vital for individuals or necessary in order to be a healthy person. But what about relationships? Well, clearly many asexual people can and do form happy and healthy relationships without sex. Also, research on sex and relationships more broadly has challenged the common assumption that sex is essential for healthy relationships.

The most recent National UK Survey of Sexual Attitudes and Lifestyles (NATSAL) found that, while sex was certainly an important part of a relationship for many people, having less sex or having sexual problems wasn't tied to relationship dissatisfaction, as many sex advisors would have us believe.[18] Similarly, a recent major study on people in long-term relationships found they had all different levels of sex in their relationships (from none at all to frequent sex) and this didn't seem to relate to how happy they were with their relationship as a whole or what kind of shape it was in. In fact people often valued other forms of emotional intimacy and/or physical closeness more highly than sex.[19]

We might also usefully challenge the assumptions in a lot of sex advice books that not only is it essential that your relationship is sexual but also that you are *in* a partner relationship in the first place, that this should be where all your sexual needs get met, and that you should fear losing it. We'll return to some of these ideas in the next chapter when we explore the diversity of ways of having sexual and non-sexual relationships.

THE MEANING OF SEX

We've covered several of the key problems with the current model of sex: it excludes people who aren't heterosexual or into PIV sex; it offers a limited view of what counts as 'proper sex' and suggests anybody who can't – or doesn't want to – conform to this is dysfunctional; and it implies everybody *should* be sexual rather than recognising that sexual desire is on a spectrum and also often fluctuates over the course of people's lives.

Biopsychosocial sex

We also saw earlier that the prevailing view tends to regard sex and its problems as primarily physiological, searching for organic *causes* and medical or physical *fixes*.[20] This tendency to focus on the biological over the psychological and social can be problematic: a biopsychosocial approach is much better at capturing everything that contributes to our sexual experience, whether positive, negative, or a combination of both. Remembering the biopsychosocial approach outlined in the previous chapter, you might want to consider the following examples.

Sex therapist Peggy Kleinplatz describes working with Ms. Smith: a client who was terrified of PIV sex and found her vagina tensed up any time she attempted it with her fiancé (she might have been diagnosed with 'penetration disorder' or 'vaginismus'). When Kleinplatz explored Ms. Smith's cultural background she found that talking about sex was completely taboo in her family, and sex was viewed as shameful, so she hadn't known what to expect from sexual relationships at all. She had a terrible first relationship with a man who pressured her to let him penetrate her and assaulted her. Talking with Kleinplatz about her experiences in that relationship helped Ms. Smith to share how powerless she felt in relationships and to explore her anger at what had happened to her. She was able to discuss ways she might take control.[21]

When I worked as a therapist myself, I had a client, Helen, who was struggling with a problem similar to Ms. Smith's. Helen found it very painful to have PIV sex because her vagina became so tense. Like Kleinplatz I tried to find out about Helen's wider world. We talked a lot about how she felt about her body. She was very negative about it, worrying her partner would be turned off by her 'muffin top' or 'cellulite' and trying to limit herself to sexual positions she'd look most attractive. We also talked about the pressures on Helen (as a woman) to always be something for other people: desirable to her partner, a good daughter for her (single) mother, doing all of the emotional labour at work. Our therapy focused on Helen tuning into herself more: learning to value herself and her goals equally to the other people in her life.[22]

These examples illustrate two things: how sexual experiences are biopsychosocial, and how different people have very different meanings around sex.

In both cases we can see how the cultural context the people grew up in was an important part of the picture: for Ms. Smith the shame and taboo around sex, for Helen the importance placed on women being desirable and being all about looking after other people. We can also see how their life experiences combined with cultural messages to give them a particular experience of sex. In Ms. Smith's case her abusive first relationship caused her fear and pain, and in Helen's case her father leaving at a young age left her with a particular fear about losing relationships. These psychosocial elements work on our brains and bodies in the ways described in the last chapter. For women in particular, cultural messages about the need to control their 'unruly bodies' can mean they get very used to tensing up – fearing the shame, for example, of people knowing they're on their period or of breaking wind in public.

You can see similar things if you compare case studies of men who lose their erections. Kleinplatz writes about one man who felt he was a failure for having to take Viagra and who was very influenced by that pressure on men to be hard and to perform which I described earlier.[23] The famous therapist Irving Yalom describes a man who had a similar problem, but for him it was much more that sex was a way of soothing himself from the fear of his impending retirement and all the things he hadn't done in his life. As retirement got closer his old way of distracting himself couldn't keep the anxiety at bay.[24] We'll return to the ways personal experiences and cultural expectations combine in influencing our erotic lives in Chapter 6.

So any aspect of sex will have different meanings for different people depending on their cultural context and their individual experiences. Just think of one sexual experience – an orgasm – and the multiple different ways people can experience it. It can be:

> a mechanical release, a demonstration of one's masculine or feminine sexuality, a relief of stress, a loss of control, allowing someone to see you at your most vulnerable, a display of intimacy, the height of physical pleasure, a transcendent spiritual experience, a performance demonstrating prowess, a giving of power to another, an exerting of power over another, a form of creative self-expression, a humorous display of our rather-ridiculous humanity, an unleashing of something wild and animalistic, a deeply embodied experience, an escape from bodily sensations and pain, and/or a moment of complete aliveness or freedom.[25]

We can understand, therefore, why some people might really want orgasms, some might prefer not to, and others might feel more neutral or ambivalent about them.

You might want to think about what sex means to you, or consider different sexual activities and experiences from this perspective. Of course, it might well be the case that each one has several different meanings – at different times or at the same time.

We've seen how – with all aspects of sex and sexuality – there are elements of our physiology, and the cultural messages we receive, which we *share* with other people, as well as experiences which are *unique* to our particular lives and bodies. For these reasons it's oversimplistic to focus on one universal cause or explanation, or treatment or fix, for any sexual experience or problem. There is no one-size-fits-all form of sex therapy or sex advice. Instead, we have to explore each unique person's *lived experience* and the meanings they have around sex. We'll talk more about these kinds of multiple meanings in the coming chapters.

SEX THERAPY

All of this has implications for how sex therapists can best work with clients – and for the kind of psychologically informed sex advice and education we might want to make available to people. From the last section you've seen it's important to explore each individual's lived experience of sex rather than assuming everyone has had the same experience of erections, penetration, orgasms, or any other aspect of sex. You've also seen it's worth remembering that sex is biopsychosocial and giving equal weight to all three aspects (biological, psychological, and social).

Focusing on pleasure rather than goals

Mainstream sex therapy has been criticised for being goal-focused rather than pleasure-focused. Gina Ogden describes it as the 'doing it' theory of sexual normalcy and the 'didja come?' theory of sexual satisfaction![26] There's a risk focusing on goals will paradoxically have the opposite effect to the one that we want. It's rather like insomnia: anybody who has suffered with this will know the worst thing you can do is to try hard to get to sleep. A similar thing is true for trying to get an erection or an orgasm. The more you try to 'achieve' it, the further away it seems to go. Sex therapists increasingly draw on mindfulness, which encourages people to 'be present' to whatever they're experiencing during sex, instead of trying to make anything particular happen: to focus on the journey rather than any destination.[27] Of course this isn't an easy task, given all the cultural pressure to have PIV sex in multiple positions and to follow a linear progression from desire through arousal to 'mindblowing' orgasms.

The NATSAL study – which I mentioned earlier – found 42% of men and 51% of women reported at least one sexual difficulty:[28] That's nearly half of the UK population who regard themselves as having a sexual problem. It's worth wondering how many of those people would see themselves in this way if we didn't have such a limited view of sex: if we expanded out the definition of what counts as sex, as well as making the aim of sex any kind of pleasure rather than reaching a certain goal which is regarded as sexual success. We'll pick up on these themes of expanding the erotic and mindful sex in Chapter 6.

If the goal of therapy is enabling erections, penetration, and orgasms, we've seen how we can easily miss what sexual problems might be telling us about the wider issues in a person's life. A penis that doesn't want to get erect or a vagina that doesn't want to be penetrated can be seen as potentially sensible: protecting us from revisiting painful experiences, for example, or from treating our bodies like machines.[29]

A focus limited to erections, penetration, and orgasm also misses the possibility of sex therapy doing something much more than re-establishing the capacity for mediocre sex. Peggy Kleinplatz suggests therapists could usefully offer their clients a range of possibilities. They might choose to do just what works to get them 'functioning', and we should honour that, but if we offer alternatives alongside this they might choose, for example, to deepen their relationships, to transform their thinking about sex, or to address their lives more widely.[30]

Sex is relational

When we're having sex with another person, or people, it's quite likely it will mean different things to each of us. For example, for the men I mentioned earlier who lost their erections, sex was all about performing or failing, being soothed or feeling anxious. For their partners, sex might have been about getting validation they were desirable, for example, or may have served as a regular ritual which made them feel secure in their relationship. So having sexual problems or stopping having sex would have different meanings for each person involved.

Without this *relational* understanding we might assume sex will mean the same thing to the other person as it does for us, or we might put extra pressure on the situation – by assuming, for example, that our sexual partner will want a certain kind of sex or by trying to persuade them because of what we want out of it. If somebody is in a relationship then it's useful to include everybody concerned in therapy because any issue is something happening *between* them, not in isolation.

Another myth about sex often perpetuated by mainstream sex advice is that partners should match perfectly in terms of both the amount of sex they want and the kind of sex they want. That's actually hardly ever the case. In any relationship there'll likely be a certain amount of overlap in extent and types of desires and also areas where there's no overlap at all. Also, because amount and type of desire fluctuate over time, this will shift and change over the course of the relationship.[31]

If we could expand our understandings of sex then it could be more possible for partners to acknowledge that these kinds of discrepancies and fluctuations are normal, and they could talk about the various options for meeting diverse sexual desires through solo sex, fantasy, or other sexual relationships, for example. However, psychologist Sandra Byers has found levels of open communication about sex in relationships are very low. People who had been in relationships for over a decade still hadn't told their partners all of their sexual likes and dislikes: They understood about 60% of what their partner liked sexually but only around 20% of what they didn't like.[32]

You might find it helpful to consider, if you have sex, how many of your sexual tastes you share with the people you have sex with. Cultural pressures and shame around sex have major implications for ensuring sex is consensual, something we'll turn to in the next chapter.

CONCLUSION

We've seen in this chapter that psychology, psychiatry, and sex therapy have tended to regard 'proper' sex as PIV intercourse leading to orgasm. People who don't experience desire, arousal/erections, or orgasms have been regarded as dysfunctional or disordered.

We've explored how this limited view of sex is present in wider culture and excludes many people, as well as placing unrealistic pressures and restrictions on those it does include. Jenny Van Hoof has found that young couples are definitely influenced by these limited understandings of sex, tending to see sex as an essential feature of long-term relationships, assuming that men need sex and that keeping a good sexual relationship going is women's work.[33]

A more open and expansive version of sex, based on the kind of research and theories we've covered in this chapter, might look something like this:

- Acknowledging it's perfectly healthy to have any level of sexual desire (from none to high and everything in between) and for this to stay the same, or change, through your life and relationships.
- Recognising all forms of consensual sex as equally valid, including solo sex and sex which involves rubbing hands or bodies together as well as various forms of penetration.
- Realising sex has different meanings for different people and tuning into our own biopsychosocial experience of sex and that of the people we're sexual with.
- Making the focus of sex 'being present' to how it feels, for everyone involved, rather than reaching any particular goal.

As with the previous chapter, an important message here is that sex is diverse. Instead of trying to compare everybody against some assumed norm, we could embrace the variation in levels and types of desire people have. This is something we'll now explore in more depth.

NOTES

1 Barker, M., Gill, R., & Harvey, L. (2018). *Mediated intimacy: Sex advice in media culture*. Polity.

2 Freud, S. (1905). *Three essays on the theory of sexuality*, trans. Ulrike Kistner. Verso.

3 Masters, W. H., & Johnson, V. E. (1966). *Human sexual response*. Little, Brown.

4 Kaplan, H. S. (1974). *The new sex therapy*. Brunner/Mazel.

5 American Psychiatric Association. (2022). *DSM-5-TR – Diagnostic and statistical manual of mental disorders*. American Psychiatric Association.

6 Kleinplatz, P. J. (2004). Beyond sexual mechanics and hydraulics: Humanising the discourse surrounding erectile dysfunction. *Journal of Humanistic Psychology*, 44 (2), 215–242.

7 Vernon, P. (2010). The race to discover Viagra for women. *The Guardian*, April 25. Available from: theguardian.com/society/2010/apr/25/women-viagra-polly-vernon

8 Hite, S. (1981). *The Hite report: A nationwide study of female sexuality*. Dell.

9 Mahar, E. A., Mintz, L. B., & Akers, B. M. (2020). Orgasm equality: Scientific findings and societal implications. *Current Sexual Health Reports*, 12 (1), 24–32.

10 Shirazi, T., Renfro, K. J., Lloyd, E., & Wallen, K. (2018). Women's experience of orgasm during intercourse: Question semantics affect women's reports and men's estimates of orgasm occurrence. *Archives of Sexual Behavior*, 47 (3), 605–613.

11 Potts, A. (2002). *The science/fiction of sex: Feminist deconstruction and the vocabularies of heterosex*. Routledge.

12 Potts, A. (2000). 'The essence of the hard on': Hegemonic masculinity and the cultural construction of 'erectile dysfunction'. *Men and Masculinities*, 3 (1), 85–103.

13 Gough, B. (2018). *Contemporary masculinities: Embodiment, emotion and wellbeing*. Springer.

14 Hille, J. J. (2023). Beyond sex: A review of recent literature on asexuality. *Current Opinion in Psychology, 49*, 101516.

15 Brotto, L. A., Knudson, G., Inskip, J., Rhodes, K., & Erskine, Y. (2010). Asexuality: A mixed-methods approach. *Archives of Sexual Behavior, 39* (3), 599–618.

16 Carrigan, M., Gupta, K., & Morrison, T. G. (2014). *Asexuality and sexual normativity*. Routledge.

17 See Young, E. (2022). *Ace voices*. Jessica Kingsley.

18 NATSAL (2013). *Sexual attitudes and lifestyles in Britain: Highlights from Natsal-3*. Available from: www.natsal.ac.uk/media/2102/natsal-infographic.pdfwww.natsal.ac.uk/media/2102/natsal-infographic.pdf. Natsal-4 was conducted between 2022 and 2024, but the findings were not available at the time of writing.

19 Barker, M. J., & Gabb, J. (2016). *The secrets of enduring love: How to make relationships last*. Penguin RandomHouse.

20 Tiefer, L. (2004). *Sex is not a natural act*. Westview Press.

21 Kleinplatz, P. J. (1998). Sex therapy for vaginismus: A review, critique and humanistic alternative. *Journal of Humanistic Psychology, 38* (2), 51–81.

22 Barker, M. (2011). De Beauvoir, Bridget Jones' pants and vaginismus. *Existential Analysis, 22* (2), 203–216.

23 Kleinplatz, P. J. (2004). Beyond sexual mechanics and hydraulics: Humanising the discourse surrounding erectile dysfunction. *Journal of Humanistic Psychology, 44* (2), 215–242.

24 Yalom, I. D. (2001). *The gift of therapy*. Piatkus.

25 Barker, M. (2011). Existential sex therapy. *Sexual and Relationship Therapy, 26* (1), 33–47. p. 40.

26 Ogden, G. (2001). The taming of the screw: Reflections on 'a new view of women's sexual problems'. In E. Kaschak & L. Tiefer (Eds.), *A new view of women's sexual problems* (pp. 17–22). Haworth. p. 18.

27 Brotto, L., & Barker, M. (Eds.). (2014). *Mindfulness in sexual and relationship therapy*. Taylor & Francis.

28 Mitchell, K. R., Mercer, C. H., Ploubidis, G. B., Jones, K. G., Datta, J., Field, N., . . . & Clifton, S. (2013). Sexual function in Britain: Findings from the third National Survey of Sexual Attitudes and Lifestyles (Natsal-3). *The Lancet, 382* (9907), 1817–1829.

29 Ussher, J. M., & Baker, C. D. (1993). *Psychological perspectives on sexual problems*. Routledge.

30 Kleinplatz, P. J. (Ed.). (2025). *New directions in sex therapy: Innovations and alternatives*. Taylor & Francis; Kleinplatz, P. & Ménard, A. (2020). *Magnificent sex: Lessons from extraordinary lovers*. Routledge.

31 Nagoski, E. (2024). I'm a sex educator. Here's the biggest myth about desire in long-term relationships. *The Guardian*, January 26th. Available from: theguardian.com/wellness/2024/jan/26/desire-myths-relationships

32 Miller, S. A., & Byers, E. S. (2004). Actual and desired duration of foreplay and intercourse: Discordance and misperceptions within heterosexual couples. *The Journal of Sex Research*, 41, 301–309.

33 Van Hooff, J. (2013). *Modern couples? Continuity and change in heterosexual relationships*. Ashgate.

4

'NORMAL' SEX

In the previous chapter we considered the implications of dividing sex into functional and dysfunctional forms. In this chapter we'll explore the other way sex has commonly been divided up: normal and abnormal kinds of sex. Remember that in the current psychiatric diagnoses and in psychology textbooks, these are the two main categories of sexual disorders: the sexual *dysfunctions* and the *paraphilias* (or abnormal sexual desires).

You saw in Chapter 2 that, since the outset of psychological thinking about sex, a key project of psychologists and other scholars in this area has been to separate normal from abnormal sex. From the early sexologists to the current American Psychiatric Association's Diagnostic and Statistical Manual of Mental Disorders (DSM-5-TR) we see lists of sexual deviations, perversions, or paraphilias. But what do we mean by normal and abnormal in this context? And is this a useful way to divide up different kinds of sex?

CONCERNING SEX

Before we go any further, it's useful to think for yourself about how you would distinguish different sexual practices. The following

DOI: 10.4324/9781003728979-4

exercise is one I developed to use when I trained therapists and other practitioners on the *paraphilic disorders*, as they're currently termed.[1]

As you read down the list, ask yourself whether or not you'd be concerned if a friend revealed they'd taken part in this activity. When you reach the end of the list, ask yourself which ones you found the most and least concerning and why. You might find it useful to note down any key concepts you find yourself using to distinguish the concerning ones from the less concerning ones.

- An individual gets a rush out of being put in terrifying situations that make him scream and cry out in fear. He engages other people to put him in a special device which will result in these effects. When his time in the device is up, his face is white and he has tears in his eyes, but he begs them to let him go through it again.
- A woman asks strangers to cause her extreme pain to her genital area. She does this regularly as she feels more attractive following the painful session. Sometimes, she'll even do it to herself. If it's done right, no permanent harm results.
- A small group of people arrange to meet in a private space in order to watch others role-playing being raped, humiliated, and tortured. They find this an enjoyable way to spend their evening.
- Two people arrange to take part in a public scene. They spend a great deal of time preparing separately in advance. On the night they dress for the occasion in clothes made of satin. Watched by a gathered group of people, they strike each other. The scene is considered successful if one of them briefly loses consciousness. The beatings are so severe they can result in permanent damage.
- A woman spends several hours preparing her appearance. She chooses from items of clothing on which she has spent several thousand pounds, all of which painfully restrict parts of her body, forcing it into an unnatural shape and making it impossible for her to function normally. Over an extended period of time she knows this will damage her permanently. However, she experiences great pleasure despite the pain.

- As part of a group ritual a man consents to an event which he knows will be gruelling, although he doesn't know exactly what will take place. During the event, among other things, he is put in an altered state of consciousness, stripped, and left alone in public.
- An individual gives his life over to his master. He won't do anything that's disapproved of under the code of rules his master has set. He won't allow himself to experience sexual satisfaction until he has undergone the procedures his master sets out as necessary, although he often finds himself in a state of arousal and wishes he could. He mostly spends time with other people who have also pledged themselves to the same master, although none of them have ever met him in person.

Drawing the line

When I used this exercise in training it generally led to useful discussions about the kinds of lines we draw to delineate concerning from non-concerning, and acceptable from unacceptable, sexual practices.

Some people say the dividing line, for them, is about whether the practice causes *damage* and whether that damage is *permanent* or *temporary*. Others distinguish between harm caused to *oneself* or to *another person*. Some say it makes a difference how *rare* or *common* an activity is or how *extreme* it seems to be. For some the *number of people* involved plays a part in their feelings about the activity, as does whether it's in the context of an *existing relationship* or with a *stranger*. People speak about lines around *illegal* activities and also around *fantasy* vs. *reality*. Others mention whether activities cause *distress* or *pleasure*.

People also frequently mention drawing lines based on whether activities are *consented* to by the people involved: whether people freely chose to get involved and whether they could give *informed consent*. For example, the group ritual often causes concern because the participant doesn't know what he's consenting to and is in an altered state. Also, members of the public may not have consented to witnessing it.

Another similar activity you could usefully try is to list all of the sexual practices that you're aware of and then try to put them on a spectrum from most acceptable to least acceptable. Draw a line on the spectrum at where you think the division is between acceptable sex and unacceptable sex. This might give you some further clues about the criteria you yourself use to delineate sex. You might also consider where you think your current understanding came from.[2]

Keep hold of your own thoughts on the exercise because we'll come back to it over the course of this chapter. You'll see psychologists, psychiatrists, and psychotherapists have also tended to use a mixture of these different concepts to decide what count as paraphilic disorders: harm, commonality, relationship context, legality, fantasy/reality, choice, and consent.

NORMAL AND ABNORMAL SEX?

Let's look now at the most recent list of paraphilic disorders, as defined by the DSM.

The paraphilic disorders

The DSM-5-TR defines paraphilias as sexual practices involving intense and persistent sexual interest other than in genital stimulation or preparatory fondling with phenotypically normal, physically mature, consenting human partners. This is the current list of the paraphilic disorders with a brief explanation of what each means:[3]

- Voyeuristic Disorder (sexually enjoying watching other people)
- Exhibitionistic Disorder (enjoying being watched)
- Sexual Masochism Disorder (finding it exciting to be humiliated, tied up, and/or to receive painful stimulation)
- Sexual Sadism Disorder (finding it exciting to do those kinds of things to another person)

- Fetishistic Disorder (getting turned on by objects or materials)
- Transvestic Disorder (becoming aroused by wearing clothes usually associated with the 'opposite sex')
- Frotteuristic Disorder (getting turned on by rubbing up against other people)
- Pedophilic Disorder (being sexually attracted to children)

So you can see several of the examples in our exercise earlier combine elements of these, particularly the first five. You might want to consider which – if any – of these might apply to you to some degree.

Up until the last edition of the DSM, simply having these sexual interests was enough to class you as being paraphilic and therefore as having a mental disorder. However, for the DSM-5 they changed this so that the interest alone did not imply a disorder. In order to be diagnosed as having a paraphilic *disorder*, you now had to meet a second criterion (criterion B) whereby it caused you some distress. This is how it was worded in DSM-5 for sexual sadism disorder, for example (the others are very similar).

> Criterion A. Over a period of at least 6 months, recurrent and intense sexual arousal from the physical or psychological suffering of another person, as manifested by fantasies, urges, or behaviours.
>
> Criterion B. The individual has acted on these sexual urges with a non-consenting person, or the sexual urges or fantasies cause clinically significant distress or impairment in social, occupational, or other important areas of functioning.

So if you occasionally find one or more of the things listed above to be sexually exciting, you wouldn't meet criterion A or B. If it was an intense and ongoing source of excitement which you were quite happy with, then you'd meet criterion A but still not be classed as having a disorder. If you had also acted on it non-consensually or it caused distress or impairment, then you'd have a paraphilic disorder, according to the DSM.

Before we go on to consider some problems with the paraphilic disorders, reflect for yourself on whether you agree that somebody who met these criteria should be classed as having a mental disorder.

Criticisms of the paraphilias

Starting with the overall definition of paraphilic disorders in the DSM – as with sexual dysfunctions in the previous chapter – you can see that, through defining abnormal and dysfunctional sex, the DSM also defines what is normal or functional sex. In this case it's genital stimulation – or preparatory fondling for genital stimulation – with somebody who is 'normal' in terms of their observable physical or biological characteristics. So again, solo sex isn't regarded as normal sex, and neither is sex with (presumably) intersex people, trans people, and possibly disabled people or people with larger or smaller body sizes than the norm (depending on how far you take the definition of 'phenotypically normal').[4] These aspects of the DSM definitions are problematic for all the reasons we considered in Chapter 3.

Perhaps the most compelling criticism people have made about the paraphilias is that they're simply a reflection of our current social mores rather than any kind of objective scientific list of pathological sexual practices.[5] This is underlined when you consider the fact homosexuality was classed as a mental disorder in the DSM until 1973 and in the World Health Organization's International Classification of Diseases (ICD) until 1992. If same-sex attraction was once a disorder and now isn't, might the other paraphilias simply be reflections of what wider culture thinks is acceptable and unacceptable sexually?

Here it's useful to return to the exercise we did before. As you went down the list, you may well have realised there's another element to this exercise, along with it being a useful way into considering the lines we draw around sexual activities. All of the activities listed are actually commonplace in mainstream culture. They describe in order: a fairground ride, a bikini wax, watching a horror movie like the *Saw* or *Halloween* series, a boxing match, wearing high-heeled shoes or a corset, a stag do or bachelor party, and the practices of many religious people.

This aspect of the exercise highlights how much *more* difficulty people tend to have with activities that are culturally non-normative or stigmatised than those that are culturally accepted. Once the 'real' activities are revealed, people often start to ask themselves whether they were *really* so bothered about damage, distress, or consent, given their concern disappears when they know what the activities actually are. Other useful comparisons to make would be play piercing in a kink context versus acupuncture or tattooing, and suspension bondage versus rock climbing.

The history of homosexuality in the DSM helps to reveal a further issue with the paraphilias. When homosexuality was first removed from the DSM it was replaced with the category of 'ego-dystonic homosexuality', which basically meant people having same-sex desires they were distressed by or which caused impairment to their lives: rather like the recent move from 'paraphilias' to 'paraphilic disorders'. The problem with this, of course, is that when you have a sexual identity or practice which is viewed as unacceptable in wider culture – to the point it was recently considered to be a mental disorder – you're not likely to feel 100% great about it! Those people who are disturbed by their kinky sexual desires – or who previously were by their same-sex desires – may well not be disordered in any inherent sense but just struggling to exist in a culture that sees them as sick, bad, or unacceptable. Of course continuing to list certain sexual practices in the DSM, even with the caveat that they're only disorders if people are unhappy with them, only perpetuates the stigma.

Finally, Charles Moser and many others have criticised the paraphilias for being muddled, unclear, inconsistent, and lacking in any basis in evidence.[6] If you think back to the reasons people gave for delineating sexual practices earlier, a mixture of these are in play in the DSM diagnoses. Some are there because they're *inevitably* non-consensual if acted upon (e.g. pedophilic disorder) or are *often* non-consensually acted upon (e.g. frotteuristic and voyeuristic disorders). With others the concern seems to be more about potential harm to others (e.g. sexual sadism disorder) or self (e.g. sexual masochism disorder). And with others, the only conceivable problem would be that the person themselves – or people in their lives – had problems with it (e.g. fetishistic and transvestic disorders). As we'll go on to see, many of the so-called paraphilias are actually very common, few are linked to mental distress in the general population, and all except paedophilia *can* be acted upon in consensual ways.

In addition to the slippage between different reasons for classifying something as paraphilic (consent, commonality, harm, etc.) there is the issue of line drawing. You may well have thought yourself that at one end of the spectrum many of the paraphilias apply to a whole lot of people. Think about how many folks enjoy watching sex-themed movies (a form of voyeurism), or wearing certain materials in sexy outfits (animal print or lace, for example – a form of fetishism), or enjoy turning people's heads when they walk into the room (a form of exhibitionism).

At what point do we decide that a person has strayed too far towards the 'abnormal' end of the spectrum? What do we mean by abnormal? And is 'normality to abnormality' the best spectrum to be using in the first place? As Moser provocatively points out, we could class heterosexual attraction as a paraphilic disorder just as much as any other sexual practice: it often involves recurrent and intense arousal which is acted on non-consensually or causes significant distress and impairment.[7]

Learning from the margins

Until recently, psychologists and related professionals who studied the paraphilias – or 'abnormal' sexual practices – have focused on *explaining* why people might engage with them: often trying to come up with universal causes of sadism, masochism, etc. as they did with same-sex attraction (see Chapter 2). In recent years, however, many of us have questioned that way of thinking, rooted as it is in cultural assumptions about acceptability, and dubious notions that any human behaviour can have one explanation which applies to everybody who engages in it (see Chapter 3).

Recent scholars and professionals have taken the radically different approach of asking what we might *learn* from those at the outer limits of human sexual experience which could be of use to everybody, rather than how we might explain them and keep them at a comfortable distance.[8] In the next two sections we'll look at what we now know about kink and about non-monogamous relationships, from this kind of psychology, and the light this shines on sexual practices and sexual relationships more widely.

KINK ETC.

Kink and BDSM are more common umbrella terms for what the DSM called sadism and masochism. Often the terms are used loosely enough that a lot of exhibitionism, voyeurism, and fetishism could fall under these umbrellas as well. BDSM stands for bondage and discipline, dominance and submission, and sadomasochism, so it covers a pretty wide range of practices.

Is BDSM a paraphilia?

Paraphilias are commonly defined as *conditions* characterised by *abnormal sexual* desires, typically involving *extreme or dangerous* activities, so let's start by examining whether BDSM can meet these criteria.

First, in order for kink to be a *condition or disorder* we'd expect kinksters to have higher rates of psychological problems than other people. Early research in this area did find relationships between being into BDSM and various forms of mental distress – until people pointed out most of that research consisted of mental health professionals writing about their clients! This is an example of the *clinician illusion* whereby practitioners assume that a practice or identity is pathological because the only people they've seen with it in their clinic have been struggling. Of course most of the people clinicians see are struggling, so that's pretty meaningless.

From the 1980s onwards, psychologists and other researchers started studying kinksters in the general population and comparing them against people who weren't into BDSM on various measures. This kind of research found no evidence that kinky people were any more psychologically unhealthy than anyone else.[9] In fact studies suggest they may even be *more* healthy,[10] with one project finding that BDSM practitioners were, on average, less neurotic, more extraverted, more open to new experiences, more conscientious, less sensitive to rejection, and reported greater well-being than a control group. Another study found no evidence for the common idea that kinky inclinations are rooted in childhood abuse and trauma, as suggested in movies like *Secretary* and *Fifty Shades of Grey*. The research found kinksters have childhoods indistinguishable from those of other people.[11]

What about being *abnormal*? Research suggests otherwise. Many studies concur that around two-thirds of people have kinky fantasies, and nearly half have acted on these at least once, over 10% on a regular basis.[12] BDSM equipment like blindfolds and handcuffs are sold in high street sex shops, and – of course – the *Fifty Shades of Grey* books and films have been international bestsellers, suggesting some degree of interest in kinky sex is commonplace: a majority rather than minority interest.

Paraphilias are about *sexual* desires, but is BDSM always sexual? For some people BDSM is about sex and for some there are orgasms involved. For other people there might be a different kind of climax (of sensation or emotion, for example) or no climax at all.[13] For some, BDSM is actually something more like a leisure activity, a sport, an art form, or a spiritual practice than what we usually tend to think of as sex.[14]

Finally, is BDSM *extreme* or *dangerous*? This is still a common depiction in mainstream media where the cops chasing down the serial killer go looking for him in the BDSM club, or the person getting into kink ends up on a slippery slope to more and more extreme activities. Some psychologists and therapists still believe these stereotypes and try to stop people from engaging in kink.[15] Actually, again, kinksters are no more likely to be abusive than anybody else. Of course, that means there will be folk in the BDSM world who will be abusive (just as there are in the general population). But it's important to remember it's no *more* likely there.

Kinksters also don't turn up in the emergency room any more than anybody else.[16] In fact, many of the activities mentioned in the exercise at the start of this chapter are far more risky and non-consensual than the many of the most common kink activities (spanking and bondage, for example). And there's no slippery slope: most people experience 'levelling off' after their initial BDSM experiences.[17] Of course some kinksters do engage in what might be considered to be more extreme practices – making kink a large part of their lives, for example, or seeking to endure high levels of pain or stimulation. However, this can be regarded as analogous with long-distance runners, rock-climbers, or other sports people. Such people also devote a lot of their lives to activities which can be very painful or risky because they're excited by what they're doing or committed to enduring it.

So we've seen none of the things that make something a paraphilia apply to BDSM as a whole. It's not associated with psychological problems, it's not abnormal, it's not necessarily even always sexual, and it's no more extreme or dangerous than many culturally accepted human behaviours. So what about turning the question around and asking what everyone else might stand to learn from kinksters?

Learning from the kinksters

People who are unfamiliar with BDSM often assume it involves a small range of things and that everyone does it for the same reason. There's a common stereotype, for example, of high-powered businessmen going to a leather-clad dominatrix to be whipped. Psychologists in the past also tried to come up with single explanations to explain all sadism or all masochism, such as it being an escape from having to be in control, as in this example. Actually BDSM includes many different practices and people do it for a multiplicity of different reasons.

For example, BDSM can include physical sensations (from feathers to candlewax to floggers), bondage (from handcuffs to rope to intricate ribbons), domination and submission (e.g. somebody waiting on somebody else, somebody ordering another person around), discipline (e.g. spanking, telling off), dressing up, and role-play (cops, pirates, medical, school, etc.). And all these things can happen separately or in combination.

For some people BDSM *can* be a way of giving up control and letting go, for others it's a fun, playful activity. It can mean taking on a different role and being somebody else for a while, it can be a form of relaxation, or it can be a way of showing strength and how much you're capable of enduring. It can help some people to explore something that scares them (such as pain or bullying), it can be a way of building intimacy with another person, or it can provide a reason for being looked after and cared for afterwards. It could mean many of these things even for the same person or on different occasions.[18]

So BDSM practices can point to ways we might expand our erotic imaginations beyond what we've learnt to regard as 'proper sex' (see Chapter 3) so we might explore different parts of the body, different sensations, different psychological states, and different relationship dynamics, we could enjoy or find exciting. BDSM can also help us to remember how every activity will have different meanings for different people. For example, someone can enjoy spanking because they like to feel humiliated, because they like the physical sensation, because they like seeing how much they can take, because they like giving up control to another person, because it makes them feel like a child, because it feels taboo, because their buttocks are a major erogenous zone for them, because it feels like an act of great intimacy with a partner, and for many other reasons or combinations of reasons.

Kinksters have come up with many useful ways to tune into what they might enjoy and communicate that to others. This is particularly helpful given what we learnt in the last chapter about how poorly people tend to communicate with sexual partners about sex. For example, 'yes, no, maybe' inventories help people to consider a wider range of sexual activities and whether they would like to try them. Traffic-light safewords or scales of 1–10 help people to check in with each other during activities about how much they're enjoying it.[19]

However, perhaps the most useful contribution from kink communities in recent years has been their increasingly sophisticated thinking on sexual consent. We'll return to this in-depth towards the end of this chapter.

NON/MONOGAMIES

One aspect of what is usually considered 'normal' sex which isn't explicitly mentioned in the list of paraphilic disorders is monogamy. Like the *sexual imperative*, which we covered in Chapter 3 and *heteronormativity*, which we covered in Chapter 2, the idea it's normal to be monogamous – or *mononormativity* – is taken so for granted that people rarely feel the need to mention it. However, it's ever-present as a background assumption, both in psychology and in wider culture.

Mononormativity

When I reviewed psychology textbooks I found that all the theories and research they included on relationships assumed these would be monogamous. Non-monogamy was only ever covered in the context of affairs or infidelity, which was represented as dangerous for relationships.[20] Relationship therapy has historically assumed the same thing: viewing married or long-term coupledom as the normal way of having relationships and trying to prevent people from acting on any attractions outside of this. Sex advice books acknowledge it's extremely common to fantasise about sex with people other than your partner and about group sex but warn against ever acting on these desires as they will inevitably result in jealousy and breakup. One of the most entertaining ways they address this paradox is to suggest that a couple having sex in front of a mirror is equivalent to having a threesome![21] Of course much mainstream media relies on *mononormativity*. How many of the plotlines in Hollywood movies, soap operas, and tabloid scandals would make sense if it was accepted that people could love – and/or have sex with – more than one person?

However, this idea that monogamy is the only way of doing relationships is deeply problematic. It's *ethnocentric*: assuming Western ideals represent the right and normal way of doing things. Globally far more societies operate on some form of non-monogamy than on monogamy.[22] Even within Western cultures the norm of monogamy obscures a reality in which secret non-monogamy is at least as common as monogamy, with rates of hidden infidelity in marriage as high as 50–70%.[23] This means we're in the position where many people are unable to have their ways of structuring their relationships legally recognised, and many others feel shame and guilt, insecurity and jealousy, in relationships which they have to pretend are monogamous when actually they're not.

Consensual non-monogamy

The few decades have seen an explosion of interest in various forms of open or consensual non-monogamy (CNM). As with asexuality, the increased potential for finding information, community, and partners online has been a large part of this increase.

When I started studying this area in the early 2000s, there were small but growing communities of swingers, gay men in open relationships, and polyamorous people.[24] The former two groups generally form couple relationships but have sex, alone or together, with people outside those relationships. Polyamory, on the other hand, involves having multiple love relationships in various forms. It's now estimated that 4–5% of people in the US and Canada engage in some form of CNM.[25]

As with kink, when some psychologists finally shifted from simply assuming that CNM was pathological or dangerous, their initial focus was on checking out and challenging many of the stigmatising stereotypes about non-monogamous people.[26] Terri Conley and her colleagues found that people generally thought a life-long monogamous relationship is most beneficial for a couple's sex life, happiness, and well-being and for any children they have.[27] However, there's evidence which challenges all of these beliefs and suggests forms of CNM can be equally beneficial. In addition to avoiding the stress involved in the deception of secret non-monogamy, researchers like Elizabeth Sheff and Maria Pallotta-Chiarolli have found many benefits of CNM for children, including the extra emotional and practical resources of having multiple parents, and role models who emphasise open communication.[28] In common with many monogamous relationships, pitfalls include the problems of attachment following breakup, and there's also the problem of stigma due to being part of a non-monogamous family in a mononormative world.[29]

Learning from consensual non-monogamy

As with kinky, asexual, and LGBTQ+ people, it can be useful to reverse the usual trend of psychologists searching for explanations for these marginalised identities and practices and instead asking what everyone might learn from the margins.

Open non-monogamous relationships have raised some important questions about the ideal form of monogamous partnership which is our current cultural norm. For example, historians and sociologists in this area have pointed out this kind of coupledom – and the nuclear family – is a relatively new phenomena.[30] In the past, people frequently entered into relationships for reasons to do with family, money, work, childcare, and so on rather than for romantic love (although this doesn't mean romantic love was never involved). In the current version there's a lot of pressure on partners to be everything to each other: best friend, lover, and co-parent; providing belonging, excitement, validation, security, and helping us meet our goals in life. Psychologist Bjarne M. Holmes has linked believing strongly in The One perfect partner to having worse relationships,[31] and psychotherapist Esther Perel has written about how difficult it is for relationships to provide warmth and stability at the same time as passion and excitement.[32]

None of this means CNM is necessarily a *better* way of having relationships than monogamy. Indeed, several authors have written about how CNM can be just as problematic as monogamy, with communities often excluding anyone outside a white middle-class norm,[33] and perpetuating rules and gender roles which can be just as restrictive as those in monogamous relationships.[34] Instead of buying into a new binary (monogamy vs. non-monogamy) and trying to figure out which one is better, it can be more useful to recognise the diversity of ways of doing relationships which are available as equally valid.

This is why I titled this section non/monogamy. Increasingly the dividing lines in this area are becoming blurred. For example, we might wonder where to situate monogamish relationships (which are somewhat open), hook-up cultures and casual sex,[35] friends-with-benefits arrangements, or soft swinging (where couples don't go as far as having sex with other people). We also need to recognise the range of different ways of being openly or secretly non-monogamous, from 'don't ask, don't tell' arrangements, to various forms of hierarchical non-monogamy (having primary and secondary partners), egalitarian polyamory (having multiple partners on the same level, for example, in a triad or family), and solo poly (being an independent individual with more than one partner).[36]

As we saw with sexual attraction and desire in previous chapters, monogamy might also be more usefully viewed on a spectrum from exclusive to open, with some people moving around that spectrum over the course of their lives and others remaining relatively fixed.[37] You might find it useful to imagine where you would put yourself on such a spectrum. If we view relationship styles as diverse rather than on some right/wrong, normal/abnormal binary then people stand more chance of being able to find an approach which works for them.

The communication which is prioritised in many forms of CNM[38] can also be helpful to people in all kinds of relationships. People in monogamous relationships often assume they share understandings of what monogamy means, but frequently they eventually find out they differ, and this can often cause a crisis.[39] It's very common for one person to think that looking at pornography or having sex online is okay while the other person thinks this is cheating, or for there to be disagreements around remaining friends with ex-partners. The idea of having open conversations about the kind of contracts and disclosures we want or don't want in relationships can be helpful for everyone.[40]

Recent work in this area is taking the ideas from CNM further, asking profound questions about how we delineate different kinds of relationships. For example, many forms of monogamy and non-monogamy still prioritise romantic relationships over friendships and other kinds of relationships. Some prioritise primary over secondary partners, or romantic partners over sexual ones, or recent forms of polyamory over traditional forms of polygamy. Relationship anarchy challenges such different valuing of relationships, and solo poly raises important questions about how singledom is culturally stigmatised.[41]

Scholars are beginning to link questions about how we value people differently in interpersonal relationships to wider current issues about the different value placed on different lives. This includes questions around immigration and refugees; austerity measures, class, and disability; racism, Islamophobia, and the #BlackLivesMatter movement; the treatment of trans people and sex workers,[42] and our relationships with other species and with the planet.[43] Alternative relating, living, and kinship patterns – beyond CNM – are being explored in relation to personal, community, and ecological sustainability.[44] We'll return to such considerations in Chapter 6.

BEYOND THE SEX HIERARCHY

Hopefully this discussion of the paraphilias in general, and kink and non-monogamy in particular, has got you thinking critically about the whole agenda of creating sex hierarchies. We've seen throughout this book how people can't be simply divided into majority and minority sexualities, functional or dysfunctional sexual experiences, or normal or abnormal sexual desires and how attempts to do so are bad both for those who are put in the inferior category *and* those who are put in the superior one.

The charmed circle

In the 1980s the sociologist Gayle Rubin presented the following diagram to illustrate the sex hierarchy that's so often perpetuated by psychology, medicine, laws, religions, and mass media (Figure 4.1).[45]

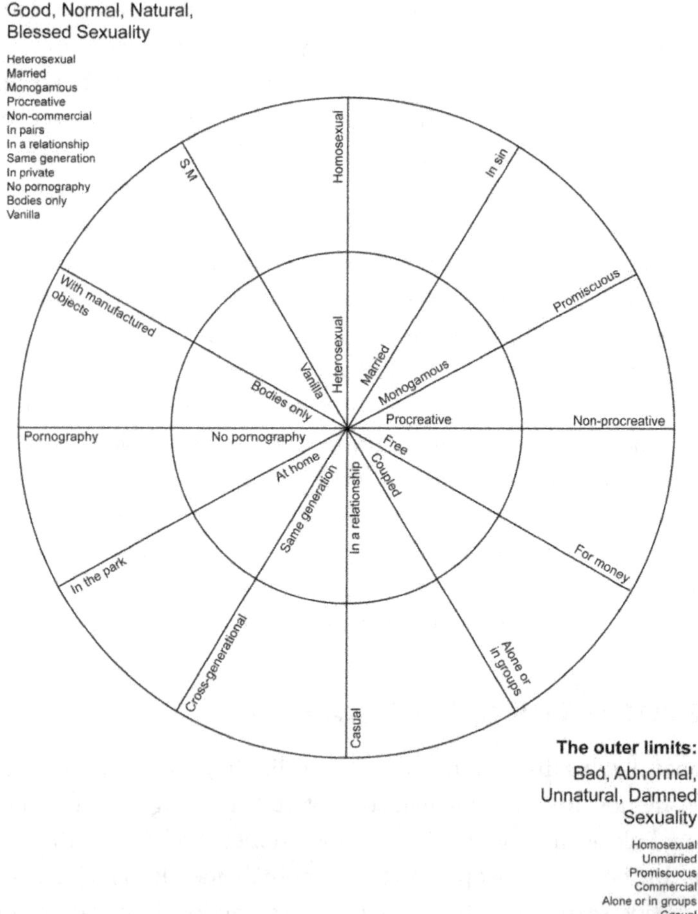

FIGURE 4.1 Gayle Rubin's charmed circle

In the inside circle of the diagram we have what she called the 'charmed circle' of sexuality. The more people's sexual relationships and practices fall into this circle, the more acceptable, good, normal, and natural they're seen as being. In the outside circle of the diagram we have the 'outer limits' of sexuality. The more people's sexual relationships and practices fall into this circle, the more unacceptable, bad, abnormal, and unnatural they're viewed as being. It's a matter of degree. Consider a straight woman who has casual sex, then add in taking payment and filming herself. Or think about same-sex marriage debates. How did gay people represent themselves in terms of these circles?

Linked to the idea of a sex hierarchy is the fear a person might fall into unacceptable sex. Rubin says we tend to see it as a slippery slope: if someone strays outside of the charmed circle a little bit they might get sucked all the way out of it. She says we fear that if we step outside 'the barrier against scary sex will crumble and something unspeakable will skitter across'. Part of the purpose of categories such as the paraphilias is to police this boundary, but it's difficult because it's built on shifting cultural sand: as you'll see in the next chapter, increasing pressure to have sex that's 'great' as well as 'normal' means many people are walking a tightrope trying to be both normal enough and sexy enough.[46]

You might want to think back to the answers you gave about where you'd draw the line between acceptable and unacceptable – or concerning and non-concerning – sex at the start of the chapter. To what extent do these map onto the kind of sex hierarchy Rubin writes about?

Before we think about alternative approaches to sex hierarchies and line drawing, let's go on a quick tangent to consider the idea of 'natural' sex. You can see from Rubin's diagram that ideal or acceptable forms of sex are often conflated with those which are natural.

What is natural sex?

It's often assumed animals only have sex for procreation – in order to pass on their genes – and this means that, whatever we want to say about sexual diversity in humans, 'natural' sex is males and females having penis-in-vagina intercourse. This isn't the case, however.

In fact, having sex at all is a recent phenomenon. Sexual reproduction in animals only began 300 million years ago and asexual reproduction is still the norm in many animals and plants, probably because it requires a lot less time and energy than sexual reproduction, and there is no risk of not finding a mate.[47] Many species who do sexually reproduce – particularly fish – also change sex during their lifetimes.[48]

It also seems other meanings of sex are at least as important as reproduction across animal species. Sex can serve to strengthen bonds between animals and within a group.[49] Many animals masturbate, and many female animals engage in sex when they're pregnant or use forms of birth control. Trans-species sex also happens, which can't result in procreation.[50] Same-sex sex happens in over 450 different species of animals across the globe, in every major animal group of all sexes, sometimes to the extent that it surpasses heterosexual behaviour in that species.[51] More than half of mammal and bird species engage in bisexual activities.

Very few animal species are monogamous, or pair-bond for life,[52] so it could be argued non-monogamy is more natural than monogamy. This demonstrates how spurious 'natural' arguments are, despite how often people deploy them to support normative assumptions and how rarely they mention them when they support non-normative ones.

Alternatives to the sex hierarchy

Authors such as Gayle Rubin and Chess Denman[53] argue that if we could get away from the desire to divide sexual practices into normal and abnormal on the basis of how culturally acceptable they are, we could open up the possibility of delineating them in far more useful ways: in relation to how much pleasure they provide and how ethical they are, for instance. Denman suggests the paraphilias should be revisited to distinguish those which are just socially *transgressive* from those which are *coercive*. She argues the latter might also more appropriately be dealt with in the realm of justice than psychology or psychiatry.[54] We'll return to some of these ideas in the next chapter.

Rubin's concept of benign variation refers to the kind of sexual diversity approach I've been emphasising throughout this book: we should regard all sex and sexuality as equally valid and acceptable so long as it's consensual for all concerned. Rubin points out that:

> most people find it difficult to grasp that whatever they like to do sexually will be thoroughly repulsive to someone else, and that whatever repels them sexually will be the most treasured delight of someone, somewhere… . Most people mistake their sexual preferences for a universal system that will or should work for everyone.[55]

We'll return to Rubin in the conclusion to the chapter. For now let's think a bit further about what's meant by this idea of sexual *consent* we've been using here.

CONSENT

Something linking BDSM communities and non-monogamous communities is the emphasis on consent. Kinksters often aspire for their play to accord with acronyms like SSC (safe, sane, consensual), RACK (risk-aware consensual sex), and CCCC (Caring, Communication, Consent, and Caution). Polyamorous and other openly non-monogamous communities often come together under the acronym CNM (consensual non-monogamy). So consent is another area where everyone might learn from the people doing their sex, and intimate, lives at the margins.

Non-consensual sex is a serious problem, with around 1 in 4 women, 1 in 6 children, and 1 in 18 men experiencing sexual violence over the course of their lives, mostly from people they know.[56] Rates of sexual violence are particularly high for trans people, particularly trans women.[57] Only around 15% of survivors of sexual violence report it, demonstrating the high levels of stigma, shame, and fear of disbelief in this area.[58]

Despite this, consent is rarely covered in any depth in sex education[59] or sex advice. In fact, my analysis of sex advice books found that the average proportion of books devoted to this topic was only just over 0%, and when it was covered consent was seen as something that was only relevant to people having kinky sex – not sex of other kinds. Consent was never given as an important reason for communicating about sex or as a topic people need to communicate about.

Quite a lot of mainstream advice explicitly suggests people – particularly women – should have sex when they don't want to have it, so they'll remain desirable to their partners and keep their relationships 'healthy'. One book claimed that women generally don't get into sex until they've been physically stimulated for a while. Another suggested that men are free to do what they want at the moment of orgasm and that they should surprise their partners by dominating them without discussing it first. This is the truly dark side of the sexual imperative because it interferes with people's ability to tune into when they do and don't want sex and means they could well be having sex which isn't consensual.[60]

Saying no and saying yes

A common understanding of consent is that sex is consensual if a person doesn't refuse someone's advances or actually say 'no'. However, psychological research in this area has demonstrated people rarely use the word 'no' in everyday or sexual interactions (e.g. being invited to the pub or being asked for sex). Instead most people follow the cultural convention of trying to let someone down gently, saying things like 'I'm afraid I'm busy tonight', 'I'm not sure', or 'maybe another time'. People generally understand very clearly that these kinds of responses mean the other person is refusing the invitation, without them actually using the word 'no'.[61]

The 'saying no' approach to consent has been criticised for assuming that consent is present until somebody takes it away. Also the emphasis is on the person receiving the sexual advances, rather than the one making them, reinforcing the cultural tendency to blame sexual assault on the behaviour of victims (what they're wearing, whether they've been drinking, etc.), rather than on perpetrators, or the wider systems and cultures they inhabit.

The 'yes means yes' or 'enthusiastic consent' model is one alternative: each partner is responsible for ensuring the other is actively enjoying the sexual activity between them, not just 'not saying no' to it, and that it's 'informed consent' so they know what they're getting into.[62] This can also be helpful when differences between people, for example, in terms of culture, class, disability, and neurodiversity, mean one person might struggle to read another's reluctance. However, the model has been criticised for suggesting that all consensual sex must be pleasurable to everybody concerned. For example, some asexual people and some sex workers consent to sex without particularly wanting it or enjoying it themselves.

Communicative consent

We can also question whether sexual consent can be established in a one-off conversation prior to sex, given that our feelings may change over the course of an interaction. Therefore, it needs to be a more active and ongoing process of communicating willingness for sex. This also gets us away from the assumed dynamic of one person actively initiating sex and another person passively accepting it, or having to refuse it.

Some have criticised the communicative consent model as being an unrealistic understanding of how sex generally progresses: ridiculing the idea that you might have to ask for permission for each touch. However, it can certainly include the more common non-verbal forms of sexual communication as well as verbal ones. Melanie Beres gives the example of undoing another person's shirt button. If they proceed to unbutton the rest of their shirt that's clear consent. If they do the button back up or clutch the gap closed, it's not.[63]

However, given the research findings on the lack of communication about sex which we touched on in Chapter 3, we have a long way to go to get to a more communicative consent model.

Consent cultures

Due to the stigmatisation of BDSM as abusive and dangerous, which we touched on earlier, for many years kink communities were at pains to insist their practices were always 'safe, sane, and consensual'. Unfortunately this had the side effect of driving the non-consensual and abusive dynamics which are present in any community underground. The consent culture movement emerged when people on the BDSM blogosphere started to discuss this more openly and to think about what might be done to prevent non-consensual and abusive sex.[64]

Many consent culture authors point out how force, control, pressure, persuasion, and manipulation are commonplace in our everyday relationships, such as in our attempts to persuade somebody to attend a social event, or in street harassment when men attempt to engage women in unwanted conversations. These authors ask whether consent is possible in sex if people are engaging in non-consensual practices within the rest of their relationships. For example, in *Fifty Shades of Grey*, Christian never hears Ana's clear 'no' about him buying her gifts, following her on holiday, and getting involved in her work. Also (as in many romantic books and films) both characters continually attempt to pressure, persuade, or cajole the other into being what they want them to be. As blogger The Pervocracy puts it, 'I think part of the reason we have trouble drawing the line "it's not okay to force someone into sexual activity" is that in many ways, forcing people to do things is part of our culture in general. Cut that shit out of your life. If someone doesn't want to go to a party, try a new food, get up and dance, make small talk at the lunchtable – that's their right. Stop the "aww c'mon" and "just this once" and the games where you playfully force someone to play along. Accept that no means no – all the time'.[65]

This links to feminist psychology research which has called attention to the normative heterosexual script we covered in Chapter 3. Nicola Gavey has pointed out how difficult consent can be under power relations where men are assumed to have a natural sex drive and to need sex, while women are not seen as actively desiring beings.[66]

Authors in the consent culture movement agree there needs to be awareness of both the circulating cultural pressures around sex and the power relations between any two (or more) people.[67] Such awareness needs to be *intersectional* (see Chapter 2), considering the impact, for example, of age, gender, sexuality, race, nationality, social position, social class, and other differences, on how possible it is for each person to say either 'no' or 'yes' to sex. As activist Pepper Mint points out, non-consensual power dynamics are so common in our schools, workplaces, and wider cultures that 'we are in fact swimming in a soup of non-consensual power dynamics, where our personal strategies are typically shaped by sets of options that can range from mildly undesirable to downright horrific'.[68]

As with research on CNM communities, this kind of work has encouraged kinksters to address the dynamics of privilege and oppression that exist within their communities and the impact this can have,[69] in some cases actively using their sexual practice to increase awareness of these matters.[70] We'll return to the impact traumatising cultures – and the personal trauma we experience within them – have on our capacity to consent in Chapter 6 as well as touching on the implications of various waves of the #metoo movement on consent conversations in the next chapter.[71]

Based on the ideas covered here, we might try to shift to a vision of consent – across our culture – which:

- Is about finding the overlap between what people actively want, rather than just not doing what they don't want
- Is an ongoing form of verbal and non-verbal communication
- Applies to the whole relationship and to all kinds of relationships not just to sex and sexual relationships
- Recognises and addresses the power dynamics which are always in play between people and which make it more difficult for them to freely consent[72]

CONCLUSION

I hope this chapter has encouraged you to think critically about all models of sex which try to divide people into normal and abnormal (or natural and unnatural, acceptable and unacceptable) on the basis of their sexual desires, identities, relationships, and practices. If we embraced a model of sexual diversity or benign variation, potentially we could put more energy into exploring what works for each individual sexually. We could work on how to ensure that the sex people do have is consensual and ethical, given just how complex and challenging this is.

Drawing on what we've covered in this book so far I've imagined a reversal of Rubin's original diagram: one which places benign variation and sexual ethics – including consent – in the centre and which relegates fixed, hierarchical understandings of sex to the outer limits. Before we go on to consider some key current debates in the psychology of sex, think about how you feel about this suggestion as an alternative to the functional/dysfunctional and normal/abnormal divisions (Figure 4.2).

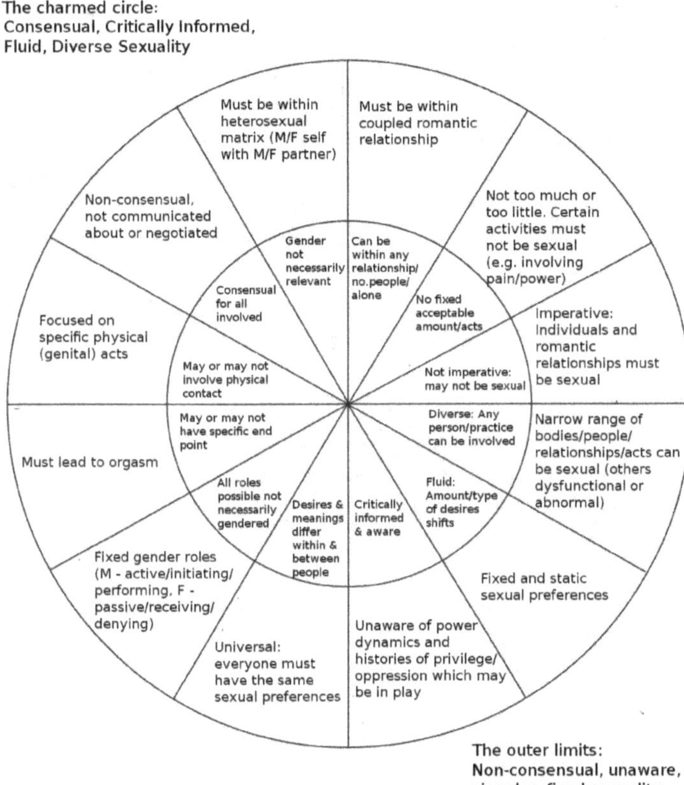

FIGURE 4.2 Rubin revisited

NOTES

1 You can read more about this and other activities in Barker, M. (2007). Turning the world upside down: Developing a tool for training about SM. In D. Langdridge & M. Barker (Eds.), *Safe, sane and consensual: Contemporary perspectives on sadomasochism* (pp. 261–270). Palgrave Macmillan.

2 There are similar exercises to this, with further exploration, in Barker, M.-J. (2018). *Rewriting the rules*. Routledge, and Barker, M.-J., & Hancock, J. (2018). *A practical guide to sex*. Icon.

3 American Psychiatric Association. (2022). *DSM-5-TR – Diagnostic and statistical manual of mental disorders*. American Psychiatric Association.

4 Barker, M. J., & Iantaffi, A. (2015). Social models of disability and sex. In H. Spandler, J. Anderson, & B. Sapey (Eds.), *Distress or disability?: Madness and the politics of disablement* (pp. 139–152). Policy Press.

5 Kutchins, H., & Kirk, S. A. (2003). *Making us crazy*. Simon and Schuster.

6 Moser, C. (2001). Paraphilia: A critique of a confused concept. In P. J. Kleinplatz (Ed.), *New directions in sex therapy: Innovations and alternatives* (pp. 91–108). Taylor & Francis.

7 Moser, C., & Kleinplatz, P. J. (2005). Does heterosexuality belong in the DSM. *Lesbian & Gay Psychology Review, 6* (3), 261–267.

8 The journal *Psychology & Sexuality* is one example of this approach and includes many articles taking a non-pathologising and affirmative stance towards the range of sexual identities and practices: tandfonline.com/journals/rpse20/about-this-journal.

9 Wilson, G. D., & Gosselin, C. (1980). Personality characteristics of fetishists, transvestites and sadomasochists. *Personality and Individual Differences, 1* (3), 289–295. Moser, C., & Levitt, E. E. (1987). An exploratory-descriptive study of a sadomasochistically oriented sample. *Journal of Sex Research, 23* (3), 322–337.

10 Wismeijer, A. A., & Assen, M. A. (2013). Psychological characteristics of BDSM practitioners. *The Journal of Sexual Medicine, 10* (8), 1943–1952.

11 Nordling, N., Sandnabba, N. K., & Santtila, P. (2000). The prevalence and effects of self-reported childhood sexual abuse among sadomasochistically oriented males and females. *Journal of Child Sexual Abuse, 9* (1), 53–63; Brown, A., Barker, E. D., & Rahman, Q. (2020). A systematic scoping review of the prevalence, etiological, psychological, and interpersonal factors associated with BDSM. *The Journal of Sex Research, 57* (6), 781–811.

12 Holvoet, L., Huys, W., Coppens, V., Seeuws, J., Goethals, K., & Morrens, M. (2017). Fifty shades of Belgian gray: The prevalence of BDSM-related fantasies and activities in the general population. *The Journal of Sexual Medicine, 14* (9), 1152–1159. More on this in Chapter 6.

13 Barker, M., Iantaffi, A., & Gupta, C. (2007). Kinky clients, kinky counselling? The challenges and potentials of BDSM. In L. Moon (Ed.), *Feeling queer or queer feelings: Counselling and sexual cultures* (pp. 106–124). Routledge.

14 Beckmann, A. (2009). *The social construction of sexuality and perversion: Deconstructing sadomasochism*. Palgrave Macmillan.

15 Kolmes, K., Stock, W., & Moser, C. (2006). Investigating bias in psychotherapy with BDSM clients. *Journal of Homosexuality, 50* (2–3), 301–324; Berman, Z. L., Mittal, M., Falconier, M. K., & Fish, J. N. (2025). Are we ready to serve? Couple and family therapists' attitudes toward BDSM and their perceived competence to help BDSM practitioners. *Sexual and Relationship Therapy, 40* (3), 695–717.

16 Kleinplatz, P. J., & Moser, C. (Eds.). (2014). *Sadomasochism: Powerful pleasures*. Routledge.

17 Nichols, M. (2006). Psychotherapeutic issues with 'kinky' clients: Clinical problems, yours and theirs. *Journal of Homosexuality, 50* (2–3), 281–300.

18 Simula, B. L., Bauer, R., & Wignall, L. (Eds.). (2023). *The power of BDSM: Play, communities, and consent in the 21st Century*. Oxford University Press; Langdridge, D., & Barker, M. (Eds.), (2007). *Safe, sane and consensual: Contemporary perspectives on sadomasochism*. Palgrave Macmillan.

19 See: Taormino, T. (Ed.). (2013). *The ultimate guide to kink: BDSM, role play and the erotic edge*. Cleis Press; Harrington, L., & Williams-Haas, M. (2012). *Playing well with others*. Greenery Press.

20 Barker, M. (2007). Heteronormativity and the exclusion of bisexuality in psychology. In V. Clarke & E. Peel (Eds.), *Out in psychology: Lesbian, gay, bisexual, trans, and queer perspectives* (pp. 86–118). Wiley.

21 Barker, M. J., Gill, R., & Harvey, L. (2018). *Mediated intimacy: Sex advice in media culture*. Polity.

22 Rubin, R. (2001). Alternative family lifestyles revisited, or whatever happened to swingers, group marriages and communes? *Journal of Family Issues, 7* (6), 711.

23 Park, W. (2019). Why we need to talk about cheating. BBC, June 26th. Available from: bbc.co.uk/future/article/20190625-why-we-need-to-talk-about-cheating

24 Barker, M., & Langdridge, D. (Eds.). (2010). *Understanding non-monogamies*. Routledge.

25 Sheff, E. (2019). Updated estimate of number of non-monogamous people in U.S. *Psychology Today*, May 27th. Available from: psychologytoday.com/gb/blog/the-polyamorists-next-door/201905/updated-estimate-of-number-of-non-monogamous-people-in-us#:~:text=In%20practical%20terms%2C%20that%20means,lesbian%2C%20and%20gay%20population%20combined.

26 Barker, M., & Langdridge, D. (2010). Whatever happened to non-monogamies? Critical reflections on recent research and theory. *Sexualities*, *13* (6), 748–772.

27 Conley, T. D., Ziegler, A., Moors, A. C., Matsick, J. L., & Valentine, B. (2012). A critical examination of popular assumptions about the benefits and outcomes of monogamous relationships. *Personality and Social Psychology Review*, *17* (2), 124–141. https://doi.org/10.1177/1088868312467087.

28 Sheff, E. (2013). *The polyamorists next door: Inside multiple-partner relationships and families*. Rowman & Littlefield.

29 Klesse, C., Cardoso, D., Pallotta-Chiarolli, M., Raab, M., Schadler, C., & Schippers, M. (2024). Introduction: Parenting, polyamory and consensual non-monogamy. Critical and queer perspectives. *Sexualities*, 27 (4), 761–772.

30 Coontz, S. (2006). *Marriage, a history: How love conquered marriage*. Penguin.

31 Holmes, B. M. (2007). In search of my 'one-and-only': Romance-related media and beliefs in romantic relationship destiny. *The Electronic Journal of Communication*, *17* (3/4), 1–29.

32 Perel, E. (2007). *Mating in captivity: Unlocking erotic intelligence*. Harper.

33 Sheff, E., & Hammers, C. (2011). The privilege of perversities: Race, class and education among polyamorists and kinksters. *Psychology & Sexuality*, 2 (3), 198–223.

34 Cassidy, M. (2025). *Radical relating*. North Atlantic Books.

35 Heldman, C., & Wade, L. (2010). Hook-up culture: Setting a new research agenda. *Sexuality Research and Social Policy*, 7 (4), 323–333; Farvid, P., & Braun, V. (2017). Unpacking the "pleasures" and "pains" of heterosexual casual sex: Beyond singular understandings. *The Journal of Sex Research*, 54 (1), 73–90.

36 Scoats, R., & Campbell, C. (2022). What do we know about consensual non-monogamy? *Current Opinion in Psychology*, 48, 101468.

37 There's a chapter exploring these spectrums in depth in Barker, M. (2018). *Rewriting the rules*. Routledge.

38 Cardoso, D. (2024). Reframing the role of communication in consensual and/or ethical (non) monogamies: A proposal for a change in academic terminology. *Open Research Europe*, 4, 167; Ritchie, A., & Barker, M. (2006). 'There aren't words for what we do or how we feel

so we have to make them up': Constructing polyamorous languages in a culture of compulsory monogamy. *Sexualities*, 9 (5), 584–601.

39 Warren, J. T., Harvey, S. M., & Agnew, C. R. (2011). One love: Explicit monogamy agreements among heterosexual young adult couples at increased risk of sexually transmitted infections. *Journal of Sex Research*, 48 (1), 1–8.

40 Barker, M. (2014). Open non-monogamies. In M. Milton (Ed.), *Sexuality: Existential perspectives* (pp. 198–216). PCCS Books.

41 Cassidy, M. (2025). *Radical relating*. North Atlantic Books; Barker, M., Heckert, J., & Wilkinson, E. (2013). Queering polyamory: From one love, to many, and back again. In T. Sanger, & Y. Taylor (Eds.), *Mapping intimacies: Relations, exchanges, affects* (pp. 190–208). Palgrave Macmillan.

42 Such themes are frequently discussed at the Non-Monogamies and Contemporary Intimacies Conference. You can access past talks here: nmciconference.com/archive/. See also: Rambukkana, N. (2015). *Fraught intimacies: Non/monogamy in the public sphere*. UBC Press.

43 For more on non-monogamies, see Vaughan, M. D., & Burnes, T. R. (Eds.). (2022). *The handbook of consensual non-monogamy: Affirming mental health practice*. Bloomsbury.

44 Rosa, S. K. (2023). *Radical intimacy*. Pluto Books.

45 Rubin, G. (1984). Thinking sex: Notes for a radical theory of the politics of sexuality. In C. S. Vance (Ed.), *Pleasure and danger: Exploring female sexuality* (pp. 267–319). Pandora.

46 Mulholland, M. (2011). When porno meets hetero: SEXPO, heteronormativity and the pornification of the mainstream. *Australian Feminist Studies*, 26 (67), 119–135.

47 Mackay, J. (2001). Why have sex? *British Medical Journal*, 322, 623.

48 Hird, M. (2004). *Sex, gender and science*. Palgrave.

49 Roughgarden, J. (2004). *Evolution's rainbow: Diversity, gender, and sexuality in nature and people*. University of California Press.

50 Hird, M. (2006). Sex diversity and evolutionary psychology. *The Psychologist*, 19 (1), 30–32.

51 Bagemihl, B. (1999). *Biological exuberance: Animal homosexuality and natural diversity*. Macmillan.

52 Barash, D. P., & Lipton, J. E. (2001). *The myth of monogamy: Fidelity and infidelity in animals and people*. WH Freeman & Co.

53 Denman, C. (2017). *Sexuality: A biopsychosocial approach*. Palgrave Macmillan.

54 Jemma Tosh's work is also helpful here as she explores attempts by psychology and psychiatry to include forms of sexual violence as paraphilias over the years: Tosh, J. (2014). *Perverse psychology: The pathologization of sexual violence and transgenderism*. Routledge.

55 Rubin, G. (1984). Thinking sex: Notes for a radical theory of the politics of sexuality. In C. S. Vance (Ed.), *Pleasure and danger: Exploring female sexuality* (pp. 267–319). Pandora. p. 283.

56 For a summary of recent figures, see rapecrisis.org.uk/get-informed/statistics-sexual-violence.

57 Crown Prosecution Service (2022). Available from: cps.gov.uk/crime-info/hate-crime/context-and-characteristics-hostility-towards-sexual-orientation-and-transgender-identity.

58 Crime survey for England and Wales (2022). Available from: ons.gov.uk/peoplepopulationandcommunity/crimeandjustice/bulletins/crimeinenglandandwales/yearendingjune2022#domestic-abuse-and-sexual-offences.

59 Whittington, E., & Hancock, J. (2024). Rethinking and redefining consent. In Louisa Allen, Mary Lou Rasmussen (Eds.), *The palgrave encyclopedia of sexuality education* (pp. 737–746). Springer Nature. Hancock, J. (2015). This is what sex education should look like. *The Guardian*, March 9th. Available from: theguardian.com/commenisfree/2015/mar/09/young-people-lessons-consent-sex-relationships-education.

60 Barker, M. J., Gill, R., & Harvey, L. (2018). *Mediated intimacy: Sex advice in media culture*. Polity.

61 Kitzinger, C., & Frith, H. (1999). Just say no? The use of conversation analysis in developing a feminist perspective on sexual refusal. *Discourse & Society*, *10* (3), 293–316; O'Byrne, R., Rapley, M., & Hansen, S. (2006). 'You couldn't say "no", could you?': Young men's understandings of sexual refusal. *Feminism & Psychology*, *16* (2), 133–154.

62 Friedman, J., & Valenti, J. (2008). *Yes means yes: Visions of female sexual power and a world without rape*. Seal Press.

63 Beres, M. A. (2007). 'Spontaneous' sexual consent: An analysis of sexual consent literature. *Feminism & Psychology*, *17* (1), 93–108.

64 Barker, M. (2013). Consent is a grey area? A comparison of understandings of consent in 50 Shades of Grey and on the BDSM blogosphere. *Sexualities*, *16* (8), 896–914.

65 The Pervocracy (2012). Consent culture. Available from: pervocracy.blogspot.co.uk/2012/01/consent-culture.html.

66 Gavey, N. (2018). *Just sex?: The cultural scaffolding of rape*. Routledge.

67 Stryker, K. (2017). *Ask: Building consent culture*. Thorntree Press; consent-culture.com.

68 Mint, P. (2007). Towards a general theory of BDSM and power. Available from: freaksexual.wordpress.com/2007/06/11/towards-a-general-theory-of-bdsm-and-power.

69 Weiss, M. (2011). *Techniques of pleasure: BDSM and the circuits of sexuality*. Duke University Press.

70 Bauer, R. (2014). *Queer BDSM intimacies: Critical consent and pushing boundaries*. Palgrave Macmillan.

71 You can read more about how understandings of consent are evolving over time in: James Alison, R. (forthcoming, 2026). From no means no to the wheel of consent: How sexual consent is evolving. *The Psychologist*.

72 For more of a working through of what it takes to be consensual, check out my 'consent checklist' zine on rewriting-the-rules.com/zines.

5

SEX DEBATES

I hope by this point in the book you've got a pretty good handle on our current cultural understandings around sexuality, what sex is, and hierarchies of sexual – and asexual – practices and relationships. You should also have a sense of some of the ways psychology has been involved in both constructing and challenging prevailing views of sex and sexuality. I hope what we've explored has shown you that psychological knowledge can never completely escape the cultural and personal assumptions of the psychologists involved in producing and presenting it. This includes the knowledge I've presented in this book, of course.

All the topics we've covered so far have been subject to fierce political and academic debates, many of which continue to this day: the rights of people with same-sex attraction, the role of sex in relationships and what constitutes cheating, which sexualities are deemed pathological or criminal, the legality of sex work.[1] Many sex-related topics have become the focus of culture wars, including LGBTQIA+ rights, sex education, and sexual violence.

In this chapter, I want to introduce you to a way of thinking critically about such debates which I've found helpful. Generally speaking, when people discuss these kinds of topics in the mainstream media, in political forums, or even at academic conferences, they

DOI: 10.4324/9781003728979-5

polarise into for and against. The underlying question driving the debate is whether this thing we're talking about is a good thing or bad thing, whether it helps people or harms people, or sometimes, as in the case of bisexuality, asexuality, or sex addiction, whether or not it's even real. It's hard not to slip into such binary ways of thinking and talking about issues because they're so entrenched in our culture.

This is a dangerous way of addressing things, however, because it leads to a lot of muddled thinking as well as to the division of people into 'us' and 'them' on the basis of their positions. And of course *we* are the enlightened, rational people with all the objective knowledge on the subject, and *they* are the irrational, biased folks basing their opinions on pseudoscience and opinion. This kind of polarisation is a key element in much human conflict,[2] and it prevents us from listening openly to others and potentially finding our way to more complex and nuanced understandings, and wise, compassionate ways of engaging with the issues that face us.[3]

In this chapter I'll keep asking the following questions. I hope you'll find them useful to apply to other issues and debates as well.

1. What are we talking about here? How is it defined? Is it one thing or many? If it's many things then we need to separate them out and address each element separately.
2. What possibilities does this thing we're talking about open up, and what does it close down? This is a more useful question than 'is it good or bad?' because it recognises most things have the potential to be both. It also keeps our focus on the *impact* of whatever we're concerned about.
3. Given the first two answers, how might we creatively engage with this thing: finding an alternative to either completely embracing it (if we find it good) or attempting to eradicate it (if we find it bad)?

Thinking back over the topics we covered through the rest of this book, I hope you'll see similar themes in the ways I've tackled, for example, sex advice, sexual practices like BDSM, consent, and so on. I find it a very helpful process to guide my thinking when journalists ask me either/or questions such as 'Is *Fifty Shades of Grey* feminist or antifeminist?',[4] 'Is the internet bad or good for relationships?'[5] or 'Is monogamy natural or unnatural?'.[6]

I'll begin this chapter by working through these questions in relation to a debate which comes around frequently: whether our culture is becoming (too) sexualised. This was the focus of a moral panic around the first time this book was published, and while it wasn't so central in the post-pandemic years of the second edition,[7] it's still useful to explore it here for many reasons. First, it's often easier to avoid immediately polarising in right and wrong positions when debates aren't so live. Second, revisiting such debates means we might learn from history when the issue comes around again. Finally, past debates around sexualisation are highly related to debates which *are* more current. For example, at the time of writing the 'gender wars' around trans included similar themes around protecting women, childhood innocence, and links between masculinity and sexual violence.[8]

Once we've explored sexualisation, I'll apply the same approach to concerns around sex and technology and then to areas which come up in relation to both sexualisation and sex tech: pornography and sex addiction.

THE SEXUALISATION OF CULTURE[9]

Sexualisation refers to anxieties that culture has become 'sexualised' and that this has had a detrimental impact on people, particularly on young people and/or women.[10] Sexualisation debates played out in politics, in the media, online, and in a number of popular books.[11]

One side of the debate argued something like: society has become hypersexual. Wherever we go we're blasted with sexual messages. Boys watch hardcore online porn from an early age, which warps their brains and turns them into sexual predators. Girls are sexualised before they're out of toddlerhood with high-heeled baby shoes, Playboy T-shirts, and Barbie or Bratz dolls. By the time they're teenagers they've bought the message from magazines and music videos that being sexy is all-important, putting them at risk of everything from eating disorders to STIs and teen pregnancy to sexual violence.

The other side of the debate emphasised choice and fun and power. It argued that we live in a time of gender equality where everyone gets to choose who they want to be, and if women want to go pole-dancing for leisure and feel empowered by dressing up sexy that's great. It claimed that sexualisation was a moral panic: the kind of thing people get worked up about every decade or so. Weren't people worrying about miniskirts and rock & roll in the same ways back in the 1950s and 1960s?

You might like to reflect on whether you remember these debates. If so, what position did you take in them? You might find it useful to go back to the three questions in the introduction to this chapter and consider them before reading on.

What do we mean by sexualisation?

I hope you can see from the overview above that part of the problem was that people used the umbrella term 'sexualisation' to refer to a multitude of different things. They were concerned with many different kinds of media and practices (music videos, lad's mags, toys, clothes, porn, sexting) and with many different possible effects (gender violence, STI transmission, sexual bullying, gender roles, child sexual abuse).

When Robbie Duchinsky and I analysed the government reports in this area we found they used the term 'sexualisation' to refer to media which do the following four things.[12]

1. Being sexually suggestive
2. Being sexist and treating women as sexual only or as sex objects
3. Encouraging children to think of themselves as adult or sexual – or inducing other people to think of children in this way
4. Glamorising or normalising deviant behaviour

When these four faces of sexualisation are conflated it makes debate difficult because disagreeing with any one of them seems like you're disagreeing with all of them. For example, a person might be concerned about girls being encouraged from an early age to be sexually desirable to boys as a key part of their identity, with very restricted ideals about what kind of appearance is attractive. However, that same person might also have real problems with attempts to censor depictions of 'deviant behaviour' given what we know about the impact of sex hierarchies (see Chapter 4) and concerns around freedom of speech. When sexualisation is presented by either side as just one thing to be for or against, it makes such positions difficult to hold and to articulate. Concern about all four aspects of sexualisation together – or dismissal of them – is presented as 'common sense'.

So it would be useful whenever we're talking about sexualisation – or anything – to define specifically *which* aspect we're speaking about and what potential effect we're trying to determine. For example, a more helpful question than 'is sexualisation harming our society?' would be as follows: 'are children watching sexual online materials and if they are, what effect does that have on them?' or 'does men's media present women in objectifying ways, and if it does, does this influence consumer attitudes and behaviour around gender and sex?'

What does it open up and close down?

Once we get specific, we can also look at each example from the point of view of what it opens up and what it closes down. Instead of assuming kids watching sexual content or women engaging in beauty routines is *either* good *or* bad, we can consider the potential they may be positive in some ways and negative in others. We can recognise the inevitable tensions and contradictions which exist in the complex world we live in.

First of all, we know that media affects different people in different ways – otherwise we'd all love and hate the same films, TV programmes, computer games, and music.[13] So we can't generalise about any particular media 'effect'. Rather, we need to explore how different audiences relate to such content, recognising some may accept what it says uncritically, others may be relatively neutral towards it, and others may resist its messages. For example, Clare Bale researched how kids related to sexual online content in various ways, including ridicule and critical analysis;[14] David Gauntlett examined how lad's mags could both perpetuate problematic forms of masculinity *and* open up possibilities for men to access more emotional expression or support.[15]

We're massively shaped by the world around us, so the sexual imagery we encounter is unlikely to leave any of us untouched. We also all filter this through our own experiences and histories in unique ways, so the same messages won't have the same impact on everybody. For this reason it's also useful for us to reflect on our own experiences and agendas in these kinds of debates. What do we bring to them? We could acknowledge that being someone who watches porn, and/or a parent, and/or a person who does or does not fit the current ideals of sexiness, all influence how we come to the debates. We might also recognise that whoever we're arguing with will likely have similar deeply personal investments in it.[16]

Creative engagement

Once we have a better understanding of what each aspect of sexualisation opens up and closes down then we're in a better position to creatively engage with it. We might find not only that a certain form of media does have a detrimental impact on young people, but also that many of them really love that media. This would lead to us thinking carefully about what they're getting out of it, how we might make media with different messages equally appealing, or enable a more critical engagement from the young people themselves.

Such mindful reflection should also help us to ask important questions about what the current concerns and debates reveal and obscure, what is included and what is excluded. For example, Robbie and I noticed that the parents who were interviewed for the report on the sexualisation of childhood were equally concerned about the impact of *sexualised* toys and clothes on their kids and the impact of *gender-stereotyped* toys and clothes. However, the report claimed the former was a grave concern with a major impact, while the latter was dismissed as inevitable, with gender preferences presented as a natural part of 'normal, healthy development of gender identity'. Again, this is an example of policy documents – and the psychological work they draw upon – constructing a certain reality. Many readings of the evidence would suggest gender stereotyping has at least as detrimental effect on children of all genders as sexualisation does.[17]

The sexualisation debate often makes a cultural assumption of childhood innocence which can be tainted by media and products. This is a problem because it can mean childhood sexuality is denied or regarded as inevitably problematic. Also children who don't follow an 'appropriate' – often heterosexual white middle class – trajectory from childhood to adulthood are stigmatised or demonised.[18] Ironically, cultural concerns over sex and childhood can mean *poorer* sex education because we become so anxious about talking to kids about sex. This often means young people are actually *more* driven to seek out sexual media in order to inform themselves.[19] With a lack of decent information, young people may be more at risk of failing to understand when they are being sexually abused or coerced. Also the huge focus on the sexual behaviour of children may mean we pay less attention to the other forms of bullying, violence, and abuse which are a major part of many young people's lives and have a devastating impact.[20] Often when such debates become polarised and inflamed, those who are most impacted – often the very people whose well-being is being argued about – become caught in the crossfire.[21]

SEX AND TECH

One focal point of concerns around sex and sexualisation has always been technology. This has burgeoned in recent years with such rapid change, including the extent to which our lives – including our intimate and erotic lives – are lived online, and advances in AI and robotics. The word 'digisexual' has been coined for a sexual attraction to – or reliance on – advanced technologies for sexual experiences. This includes relationships with machines, virtual reality, and technologically mediated sex toys, as well as tools which facilitate or enhance sexual experiences with human partners.[22]

In this section I'll explore two of these areas to consider how we might engage differently with debates around sex and tech, away from polarised arguments about whether it's 'good' or 'bad' and the kinds of blanket freedoms or restrictions which tend to flow from these.

I'll just touch on these briefly as I'm aware that the technological and cultural landscape when you read this will likely already look very different to how it appears to me at the time of writing. Then I'll focus the rest of the chapter on two key areas of concern which often come up in conversations about sex and tech: access to pornography and the potential that people might become addicted to it.

So let's explore a couple of current common areas of debate, using the structure of asking: 'what do we mean by it?', 'what does it open up and close down?', and 'how might we creatively engage with it?' I've based each of my answers on what I've learnt from colleagues who study and practice in these areas, referencing a couple of key ones who you can go to if you want to find out more. Of course your answers to these questions may well be different to mine.

Smartphones mediating our sex lives

- *What do we mean by it?* People are living their intimate lives through their smartphones in all kinds of ways: meeting people via dating and hook-up apps, engaging in sex work via internet subscription services, sexting, sharing erotic fan fiction, facilitating long-distance relationships or having whole relationships via social media or gaming platforms, sharing erotic images of themselves as flirtation or sexual harassment. Each of these needs careful consideration in itself, rather than lumping it together with all the others.

- *What does it open up and close down?* Picking just one of these, we might ask – as Kevin Guyan did in his research[23] – what's opened up and closed down by the proliferation of dating app categories for the different kinds of sexualities and genders we might identify with ourselves and find desirable in others. Guyan highlights how, while burgeoning numbers of categories (grey-A, heteroflexible, sapiosexual, twink, etc.) can ensure that more people are included in these apps, and help us to find people who are a good fit for us, they can also lead to us shaping ourselves to what dominant culture currently deems desirable, and becoming stuck in identities and expressions which don't feel authentic or are hard to sustain physically and/or psychologically. At worst, such categories legitimise people identifying their desires in racist, ableist, and otherwise discriminatory ways, reinforcing a culture where certain attributes are deemed more attractive than others.[24]
- *How might we creatively engage with it?* Guyan considered the role of burgeoning dating app categories in enabling more people to find where they fit, outside of heteronormative and cisnormative categories of sex and gender. However, he highlights the need to think carefully about algorithms to ensure apps don't limit us to only engaging with people they assume we'd be interested in, based on these categories. Beyond addressing algorithms – and other aspects of technology – support is needed to navigate the painful contradictions between an online world which seems to encourage us to find sex and gender expressions beyond binaries, and wider cultures and politics where these things are being defined far more rigidly, and resources are being withdrawn from those who want, or need, to explore them.[25]

Online social movements

- *What do we mean by it?* Recent years have seen many online social movements which relate to sex and sexuality, including survivor-led movements for increasing awareness of rape, sexual assault, abuse, and harassment, and movements for addressing the struggles that many people – particularly men – have in finding sexual and intimate connections. Even within these movements, it's important to delineate which one we're talking about as well as mapping how they change over time. For example, the original #metoo movement started by Tarana Burke in 2006 was significantly different to the version which emerged when the hashtag went viral in 2017.[26] Similarly, the Involuntary Celibacy Project, created in the late 1990s to provide mutual support for people who were lonely and struggling to find partners, is very different to recent forms of incel subculture whose online discourse is characterised by antifeminism, dehumanisation of women, resentment, self-loathing, a sense of entitlement to sex, and rape culture.[27]
- *What does it open up and close down?* Taking these two examples, we might explore what #metoo going viral opened up in terms of highlighting how common sexual assault and abuse were, helping people to recognise their experiences as abuse, enabling support, and connecting sexual violence to men in positions of power in particular. And we might also reflect on how – severed from its Black feminist origins – #metoo risked focusing on taking down certain individuals rather than creating systemic change, often centring particular survivors (particularly young white women) which made it hard for people from other demographics to recognise themselves or speak out.[28] Similarly, we might reflect on the need for supportive men's movements at a time when dominant forms of masculinity are often so toxic, including to men themselves, and value the way these can equip men with relational and emotional skills.[29] At the same time we might be alert for the ways such movements can end up

blaming those with less power for men's suffering, rather than critiquing dominant cultures and politics.[30]

- *How might we creatively engage with it?* To me, these examples both point to the need for joined up movements and solidarity, rather than separate movements based on our own personal struggles. This takes us back to intersectionality (see Chapter 2) which stresses our interdependence and interconnectedness (see Chapter 6). What might survivor movements look like which (re) joined up with abolitionist struggles in their recognition of the deep injustices in the criminal justice system?[31] Perhaps finding different approaches than policing and punishing perpetrators would enable more people to speak out about having behaved non-consensually – or having non-consensual desires. Such people could get then access the support they need not act out of those places, and survivors could have the reality and impact of the violence against them fully acknowledged (see Chapter 6). Relatedly, what might men's movements look like which appreciated that the social structures and systems which make it difficult for them to express their vulnerability and access support or pleasure are the same ones which expose women to the risk of sexual violence and deny trans and non-binary people rights and recognition?

Hopefully these examples illuminate why blanket approaches to such issues are often problematic. For example, simply restricting young people's access to sex-related content online can mean less unwanted exposure to sexual imagery, including sexual bullying and harassment. However, it also restricts their access to vital sex education, to communities and resources for people with their sexual identity, and to potentially safer exploration of their burgeoning sexualities in creative, careful ways such as reading and sharing fan fiction[32] or engaging in erotic message exchanges. With AI, polarised debates are problematic because two opposite positions are often simultaneously true: 'AI is both emotionally intelligent and tone deaf. It is both a glorified text predictor and a highly creative partner. It is costing jobs, yet creating them. It is dumbing us down, but also powering us up'.[33]

Feel free to pick your own example, from debates around sex and technology which are going on as you're reading this book, to see how working through these questions might be useful. For example, you could explore people having erotic encounters – or relationships – with AI, bots or machines, or sex toys (see Power & Waling, 2024 for more information)[34].

Now I'll explore, in more depth, common concerns within sexualisation and sex/tech debates: porn and sex addiction.

PORN PANIC

Before we go on, you might like to think about your own position on porn. Is it something you've engaged with? What views do you have on porn in general and on different forms of sexual media? Again you might like to reflect on the three questions in the introduction to this chapter in relation to porn.

Mainstream psychology has engaged with the impact of pornography many times over the years.[35] However, it often runs into methodological problems. There's no one perfect kind of research we could do to tell us the effects of reading or watching porn. Some psychologists have shown students porn in a lab and studied whether they give somebody more electric shocks or score differently on measures of sexist attitudes afterwards. But there are issues about whether the findings of such studies would apply to other kinds of people in real-world contexts. Others have investigated whether countries with more porn have higher levels of sexual violence, for example. But even if they did we can't be sure whether the porn caused the violence, or violent people bought more porn, or whether some other aspect (such as wider cultural norms around masculinity)[36] was responsible for both the higher interest in porn and the sexual violence. It's the classic correlation-doesn't-equal-causation problem.[37] Other psychologists have asked perpetrators of sexual violence about their usage of porn, but of course they might not give honest answers, and – again – we can't be sure whether those who looked at porn did so *because* of their tastes in sexual violence or whether it *caused* that.

When psychologists review the results of all of these different kinds of research, the results are inconsistent. Some lab experiments do show effects of *violent* pornography on men's attitudes towards women and on aggression, but other forms of porn have no effects or even opposite ones.[38] Countries where porn has become more easily accessible generally show no increase in sex crimes.[39] Sex offenders often had less, and later, exposure to porn than other kinds of offenders.[40]

What do we mean by porn?

As before, it's important to start by defining what we mean by porn.[41] Some of the inconsistencies in the research findings might be explained because psychologists have included different things as porn, in addition to studying their impact on different groups of people and in different contexts.

The legal definition of pornography in Britain is materials 'produced solely or principally for the purposes of sexual arousal'.[42] Obviously this includes a vast array of different things, from photo shoots in magazines, to *Fifty Shades of Grey*, to mainstream porn clips, to violent sexual images, to sexting,[43] to erotic fan fiction, to feminist porn vids,[44] and a great deal more. It's often said that the line between erotica and porn is very much dependent on the tastes of whoever is doing the defining.[45] Even if we focus in on violent or extreme pornography[46] it's very difficult to pin down. Current definitions could include images of consensual BDSM practices akin to acupuncture, for example (see Chapter 4), but not 'torture porn' movies like the *Saw* series because those are mainstream films which don't explicitly aim to sexually arouse.

As lawyer Myles Jackman[47] points out, context can mean that something which wasn't intended as porn becomes so (e.g. if the torture scene from *Casino Royale* was edited together with similar scenes from other movies) or that something which was pornographic ceases to be so (e.g. viral porn movie clips which are circulated for shock or humour value rather than to produce sexual arousal).[48]

What does it open up and close down?

Just as there are many different kinds of porn, people often engage with porn for many different reasons.[49] The meanings porn has for people, and the ways they engage with it, may well be very important in determining whether they find it to be a positive, negative, or neutral thing in their lives or all of these things.

Research suggests, for example, that those who engage with online porn have both more relationship problems *and* better sexual knowledge and attitudes.[50] Aleksandra Antevska and Nicola Gavey's in-depth interviews with young men who viewed mainstream porn found that most of them downplayed the sexism involved in the standard dominant men/submissive women script with its focus on male sexual pleasure and extreme sexual acts. However, a minority of the men critically reflected on the ethical dilemmas posed by what they were viewing.[51] Rachael Liberman's conversations with producers and consumers of feminist porn found that they saw it as a more explicitly ethical alternative to mainstream porn, which helped them to actively explore different sexual practices and identities.[52]

Alan McKee and his colleagues found that porn helps young people to develop several key aspects of healthy sexual development[53] such as learning what they might enjoy, self-acceptance, open communication with partners, and feeling that sex can be pleasurable and joyful rather than aggressive and coercive (depictions of joyless sex are not popular with most porn viewers). Porn is, however, also bad at promoting the healthy sexual development features of consensual negotiation of sex, safer sex, public/private boundaries, and relationship skills.[54]

Creative engagement

This more complex and nuanced kind of research gives us some pointers about how we might creatively engage with the existence of pornography. For example, what might we learn from the young men who *do* engage critically with mainstream porn about what encourages them to do so, and from producers and consumers of feminist and ethical porn about what is possible in sex media?

The research of McKee and his colleagues highlights the fact that good sex and relationship education (SRE) and advice are essential for plugging the gaps in the areas where porn is poor at promoting healthy sexual development. Unfortunately, though, despite calls for something different,[55] SRE frequently focuses on safer PIV sex, rather than on gender and sexual diversity, and issues such as consent, communication, relationships, and pleasure, which is what young people are often most concerned with.[56]

As with sexualisation, we can ask useful questions about the focus on porn as an explanation for various problems by mainstream media and politicians, in the criminal justice system, and by psychology. What does this focus on porn obscure or exclude?

As with many examples of blaming specific media,[57] porn *can* be a handy cultural scapegoat. It enables us to focus on an evil outside force, rather than asking more uncomfortable questions about the role of structural inequalities (in which we're all implicated) in crime.[58] It also focuses attention away from the problematic ideas about sex, gender, and violence which are around us all of the time[59] in mainstream media and in everyday conversations.[60] For example, instead of concentrating on porn we might worry just as much about the impact of the messages in sex advice about the kind of sex people *should* be having (see Chapters 3 and 4), in women's magazines about how women should look and behave,[61] and in men's media where rape myths are frequently perpetuated.[62] We could also usefully examine the problematic ideas that are present in court cases[63] and political debates[64] themselves. To tackle the problems of sexism, narrow representations of sex, and sexual violence and abuse, we need to cast the net a lot wider than porn alone.

SEX ADDICTS

Another recent concern which comes up in debate about sexualisation, and sex and technology, is sex addiction: the idea that many people (especially men) are becoming addicted to sex. This is argued to be causing relationship problems and breakdown, financial difficulties and job losses, and rises in STIs and unplanned pregnancies.[65] There are particular anxieties that addiction to internet porn and online sex are on the increase and that these are addictive in a way similar to drugs and alcohol, altering brain structure and chemistry such that people can no longer gain pleasure from other forms of sex.

While lack of agreement in this area means sex addiction, or 'hypersexual disorder', has not been added to the DSM list of sexual dysfunctions (see Chapter 3),[66] many psychologists and psychotherapists offer expertise in sex addiction and services to treat sex addicts. Sex addiction is listed as a common sexual problem by recognised sex and relationship therapy organisations.

What do we mean by sex addiction?

This proposed diagnostic term, 'hypersexual disorder', gives us a clue to the meaning of sex addiction. If 'hypoactive sexual desire disorder' refers to desire being too low (see Chapter 3), then 'hypersexual' refers to it being too high. Paul Joannides argues psychiatrists and psychotherapists are basing their ideas on a 'Goldilocks' amount of sex (not too little and not too much). But the 'appropriate level' varies greatly between individual practitioners and theoretical approaches. He gives the example of one study which regarded masturbation due to loneliness as a sign of sexual addiction. He asks, what level of loneliness is acceptable in life? And who determines the 'correct' reasons for masturbation?[67] Some people have suggested that the Goldilocks amount of sex is generally the amount of sex the practitioner is having themselves!

Some more insights into what therapists mean by sex addiction can be found if we look at the definitions given by major sex therapy bodies. One includes the following list:

While many people with no sexual behavioural problem may take part in the activities below, signs of sexual addiction may include:

- Compulsive masturbation (self-stimulation)
- Multiple affairs (extra-marital affairs)
- Multiple or anonymous sexual partners and/or one-night stands
- Consistent use of pornography
- Unsafe sex
- Phone or computer sex (cybersex)
- Sex work or use of sex workers
- Exhibitionism
- Obsessive dating through personal ads
- Sexual harassment
- Voyeurism (watching others) and/or stalking
- Law breaking[68]

Having read Chapter 4 I hope you'll immediately see some issues with this list, along the lines of the ones we discussed concerning the criteria for paraphilic disorders. Here we are first given the proviso that these things are only a problem if they're *experienced* as problematic. However, as we know, there's the dangerous feedback loop that the very fact of listing behaviours as signs of sex addiction or disorder stigmatises them further, meaning people are more likely to feel ashamed and bad about them. There's also the usual slippage between transgressive and coercive practices here, and a sense that 'outer limits' sexual practices are far more likely to be addictive than those in the 'charmed circle'. The link with addiction further stigmatises groups and practices which are already marginalised enough in our culture. Little thought is given to the potential impact of this on those who engage in solo sex, online sex, non-monogamy, or sex work. Critics have also pointed out that some of these practices are particularly common among gay men, so there's a real risk this becomes a new way of pathologising them, now homosexuality itself is no longer classed as a disorder.[69]

Finally, it's clear that, like sexualisation and porn, sex addiction is an umbrella term which covers many different things. Does it make sense to lump together people who continually seek out the hot intensity of new relationship energy (sex and love addiction), with people who spend long periods masturbating, with those who have many casual sexual partners, with those who find webcam sex online compulsive, with those who are having an affair, and so on?

What does it open up and close down?

There are many reasons to be cautious about diagnosing somebody as a sex addict. In addition to the issues of coherence, we might question whether there is *really* any increase in sex addiction or whether it's more an increase in the popularity of the term and people being encouraged to be concerned about these behaviours.[70] Remembering back to Chapter 2 we might point out that *everything* we do influences our brains – so insisting that an effect is 'real' because it causes brain changes is questionable.[71]

It's certainly the case that some people *do* experience problems with their sexual desires and practices, feeling compelled to spend a lot of time and energy on forms of sex which interfere with other aspects of their lives, or which they feel uncomfortable or distressed about, or which put them at risk in various ways.

If somebody regards themselves as a sex addict, it's important to clarify what this person *means* by sex addiction. The second of our questions is also useful: what does the label of sex addict open up and close down for them? It could be just as disempowering to dismiss a person's sense of themselves as a sex addict as it would be to accept it without question. If, instead, we explore the pros and cons of such a label people can hold it more openly: recognising the struggles they're having but not grasping the idea that they must be 'sex addicts' as some kind of fixed identity.

When I worked as a therapist, I spoke with clients who said the label 'sex addict' gave them the sense that there was something real going on for them, that they weren't simply to blame for it, and that there were other people struggling in the same way who they could get support and understanding from. However, they often worried that the label of 'sex addict' would stick to them; that being a sex addict meant there was no possibility for change; that it didn't recognise the uniqueness of their experience which was not identical to everyone else's; and that if they were diagnosed in this way people wouldn't acknowledge what it was which was so compelling and important for them about the sex they were pursuing – even if it did cause them problems.[72]

Creative engagement

When creatively engaging with a person who's struggling with 'sex addiction' it's important to discuss the cultural messages they've received about sex. Is this thing a problem because it's upsetting them, or is it a problem because society sees it as 'bad' or because other people in their life have a problem with it? Obviously these things aren't always easy to disentangle.

It's also useful to keep 'opening up and closing down' in mind. While what they're doing is obviously distressing (given they're seeking help for it), it also must be giving them something too, in order to be so compelling to them. We might usefully explore both the losses and the gains involved. As with the other kinds of sexual struggles we covered in Chapter 3, a key thing here is to explore the multiple *meanings* 'sex addiction' has for the individual person. For example, I worked with two young men who spent a lot of their time on online sexual encounters. However, what they got out of it couldn't have been more different. For one it was a soothing activity where he could escape from the tough realities of his life into a kind of black hole where he didn't have to feel anxious. For the other, it was the place he felt most alive and awake: cybersex enabled him to unleash a confident, dominant persona he couldn't let himself be in the rest of his life and to express the kind of creativity which wasn't possible in his dull job.

Some conventional 'treatments' for addiction involve abstinence: people simply stopping the problematic behaviour. This risks not allowing people to become aware of what their behaviour *means* to them and what they *gain* from it. Also people often end up swinging from complete abstinence to going back to the compulsion – and feeling terrible about it.[73] The mindfulness idea of 'being present' is useful here. Instead of losing ourselves in the behaviour or trying to avoid it completely, we can engage in it in a slower, more self-aware way, reflecting afterwards about what was so compelling about it for us.[74]

We'll consider the meanings of sexual desires and fantasies in more detail in Chapter 6 as well as how we might cultivate more mindful, conscious approaches to sex in general.

CONCLUSIONS

This chapter might have given the impression that the answer to all the fraught, polarised debates which face us around sex – and everything – is simple: just get everyone to work their way carefully through the kinds of questions I suggest here, and this will open things out and lead us to creative ways forward which keep everyone's needs in mind. Obviously it isn't as straightforward as this, otherwise such things wouldn't escalate into all-out culture wars, harming those on both sides, and particularly those caught in the crossfire.

As you read the chapter you might have noticed yourself able to work through the three questions calmly and clearly around some topics, while – with others – you felt more tense or confused while reading them, maybe thinking that surely there was an obvious right and wrong in that case. Such experiences give us a clue about what's missing in attempts to rationally address – and research and theorise about – these kinds of areas: feelings.

Polarised debates, moral panics, and culture wars frequently happen around topics which bring up unbearable emotions for people. The urge to prove your way of seeing things right, and others wrong, is one way of avoiding monstrous feelings which threaten to overwhelm us.

This is understandable when you think about how, underlying all these issues, are huge existential themes of life and death, safety and danger, belonging and exclusion, freedom and oppression, who is included in the category of human, and who isn't. Relatedly, such topics often tap into areas of personal trauma where we, ourselves, have been under threat, rejected, or abused, including early in life when we were particularly vulnerable. We may not always be consciously aware of such links, but this is a big part of why, for example, someone might want to do anything to eradicate images of women being objectified, to protect the innocence of children like they once were, or to punish certain kinds of perpetrators; why they may be highly motivated to ensure that everyone is free to experience certain kinds of pleasure, to deny that certain kinds of abuse or oppression exist or have an impact, or to say whatever they like.[75]

When a debate is hot and polarised for us, it often connects with areas of cultural and personal trauma. In order to escape the unbearable feelings this brings up – like shame, rage, terror, and loneliness – we may intellectualise to avoid such feelings, attack-out to prove ourselves right and others wrong, withdraw from any conversation that risks exposing us to such conflicts, or attack-in and shame ourselves for not doing enough or for being one of the kinds of people others are attacking, perhaps finding ourselves agreeing with whoever we're with in order to appease them.

In the final chapter of this book we'll now turn to the role of such unconscious processes – and trauma – in sex.

NOTES

1 Smith, M., & Mac, J. (2018). *Revolting prostitutes: The fight for sex workers' rights*. Verso Books.
2 The *5 Steps to Tyranny* documentary is a really accessible overview of the psychological research in this area, summarised in this article, and available online: theguardian.com/media/2000/dec/19/tvandradio.television1
3 Alex Iantaffi and I work through this in more detail in our book: Barker, M. J., & Iantaffi, A. (2019). *Life isn't binary*. Jessica Kingsley.
4 Barker, M.-J. (2012). 50 shades feminist. Available from: http://rewriting-the-rules.com/2012/07/04/50-shades-feminist/.
5 Barker, M.-J. (2014). The internet and relationships. Available from: http://rewriting-the-rules.com/2014/11/17/the-internet-and-relationships/.
6 Barker, M. (2013). So monogamy works for some animals. Doesn't mean it's 'natural' for us. Available from: www.theguardian.com/commentisfree/2013/jul/30/monogamy-animals-evolutionary-research.
7 In fact there were even concerns that people, including young people, weren't being sexual *enough*: Masoudi, M., Maasoumi, R., & Bragazzi, N. L. (2022). Effects of the COVID-19 pandemic on sexual functioning and activity: A systematic review and meta-analysis. *BMC Public Health*, 22 (1), 189; Fry, H. (2023). A 'failure to launch': Why young people are having less sex. *Los Angeles Times*, August 3rd. Available from: https://www.latimes.com/california/story/2023–08-03/young-adults-less-sex-gen-z-millennials-generations-parents-grandparents.
8 I'll return to this towards the end of the chapter and have applied a similar approach to this in: Barker, M. J., & Ryan-Flood, R. (2023). The gender wars and difficult conversations about trans: An interview with Meg-John Barker. In Róisín Ryan-Flood, Isabel Crowhurst, Laurie James-Hawkins (Eds.), *Difficult conversations* (pp. 11–26). Routledge.
9 This section is drawn from *The Sexualization Report*: an online resource colleagues put together of information and research about sexualisation: thesexualizationreport.wordpress.com. The website onscenity.org also brings together a number of writers on this topic. And badsexmediabingo.wordpress.com draws on this work to highlight problematic media depictions of sex.

10 APA Report. (2007). *American Psychological Association, task force on the sexualization of girls*. Available from: apa.org/pi/women/programs/girls/report; Bailey, R. (2011). *Letting children be children*. Department for Education. Available from: gov.uk/government/publications/letting-children-be-children-report-of-an-independent-review-of-the-commercialisation-and-sexualisation-of-childhood; Buckingham, D., Willett, R., Bragg, S., & Russell, R. (2010). *External research on sexualised goods aimed at children*. Report to Scottish Parliament Equal Opportunities Committee, SP Paper 374; Byron, T. (2008). *Safer children in a digital world: The report of the Byron Review 2008*. Victoria, BC: DCSF' Papadopoulos, L. (2010). *Sexualisation of young people review*. Available from: dera.ioe.ac.uk/id/eprint/10738/1/sexualisation-young-people.pdf; Rush, E., & La Nauze, A. (October 2006). *Corporate paedophilia: Sexualisation of children in Australia*. Australia Institute.

11 e.g. Levin, D., & Kilbourne, J. E. (2008). *So sexy, so soon: The new sexualized childhood and what parents can do to protect their kids*. Ballantine Books; Sarracino, C., & Scott, K. M. (2008). *The porning of America: The rise of porn culture, what it means, and where we go from here*. Beacon Press.

12 Barker, M., & Duschinsky, R. (2012). Sexualisation's four faces: Sexualisation and gender stereotyping in the Bailey Review. *Gender and Education*, 24 (3), 303–310.

13 Hoyle, A. (2012). Should we panic about pornography? Available from: www.tes.com/article.aspx?storycode=6287772.

14 Bale, C. (2011). Raunch or romance? Framing and interpreting the relationship between sexualized culture and young people's sexual health. *Sex Education*, 11 (3), 303–313.

15 His chapter on this in the following book is helpful, and the book as a whole is a good one if you're interested in media impact more broadly. Gauntlett, D. (2008). *Media, gender and identity: An introduction*. Routledge.

16 Gergen, K. (2015). *An invitation to social constructionism*. Sage.

17 Fine, C. (2010). *Delusions of gender: The real science behind sex differences*. Icon Books.

18 Egan, R. D. (2013). *Becoming sexual: A critical appraisal of the sexualization of girls*. John Wiley & Sons.

19 Alldred, P., & David, M. E. (2007). *Get real about sex: The politics and practice of sex education*. Open University Press.

20 Read, J., & Bentall, R. P. (2012). Negative childhood experiences and mental health: Theoretical, clinical and primary prevention implications. *The British Journal of Psychiatry*, 200 (2), 89–91.

21 For example, see Yarrow, E. (2024). Gendering innocence: An empirical inquiry into the lived experience of gender incongruence in childhood. *Children & Society*, 38 (6), 1984–2002.

22 Neves, S. (2022). *Sexology: The basics*. Routledge; Attwood, F., Hakim, J., & Winch, A. (2017). Mediated intimacies: Bodies, technologies and relationships. *Journal of Gender Studies*, 26 (3), 249–253.

23 Guyan, K. (2025). *Rainbow trap: Queer lives, classifications and the dangers of inclusion*. Bloomsbury Publishing. See also: theconversation.com/dating-app-categories-could-be-shaping-you-more-than-you-know-256368.

24 I work through this here: rewriting-the-rules.com/sex/sapiosexuality.

25 Butler, J. (2025). *Who's afraid of gender?* Random House.

26 Gregory, T. (2023). Tarana Burke discusses her me too movement, Hollywood's hashtag co-opting of it. *University of Chicago News*, March 29th. Available from: news.uchicago.edu/story/tarana-burke-discusses-her-me-too-movement-hollywoods-hashtag-co-opting-it.

27 Kassam, A. (2018). Woman behind 'incel' says angry men hijacked her word 'as a weapon of war'. *The Guardian*, April 26th. Available from: https://www.theguardian.com/world/2018/apr/25/woman-who-invented-incel-movement-interview-toronto-attack.

28 Phipps, A. (2020). *Me, not you: The trouble with mainstream feminism*. Manchester University Press.

29 O'Neill, R. (2018). *Seduction: Men, masculinity and mediated intimacy*. John Wiley & Sons.

30 Copeland, S. J. (2025). *The male complaint*. Polity.

31 Davis, A. Y., Dent, G., Meiners, E., & Richie, B. (2022). *Abolition. Feminism. Now*. Penguin.

32 Popova, M. (2021). *Dubcon: Fanfiction, power, and sexual consent*. MIT Press.

33 Connock, A. (2025). I got an AI to impersonate me… *The Conversation*, August 18th. Available from: theconversation.com/i-got-an-ai-to-impersonate-me-and-teach-me-my-own-course-heres-what-i-learned-about-the-future-of-education-262734.

34 Power, J., & Waling, A. (2024). *Tech, Sex and Health: The Place of New Technologies in Sex, Sexual Health, and Human Intimacy*. Routledge.

35 Barker, M. (2014). Psychology and pornography: Some reflections. *Porn Studies*, 1 (1–2), 120–126.

36 Murnen, S. K. (2015). A social constructivist approach to understanding the relationship between masculinity and sexual aggression. *Psychology of Men & Masculinity*, 16 (4), 370–373.

37 Infographic of the day (2014). Hilarious graphs prove that correlation isn't causation. Available from: fastcompany.com/3030529/hilarious-graphs-prove-that-correlation-isnt-causation.

38 Mellor, E., & Duff, S. (2019). The use of pornography and the relationship between pornography exposure and sexual offending in males: A systematic review. *Aggression and Violent Behavior, 46*, 116–126.

39 Diamond, M., Jozifkova, E., & Weiss, P. (2011). Pornography and sex crimes in the Czech Republic. *Archives of Sexual Behavior, 40* (5), 1037–1043.

40 Ferguson, C. J., & Hartley, R. D. (2009). The pleasure is momentary… the expense damnable?: The influence of pornography on rape and sexual assault. *Aggression and Violent Behavior, 14* (5), 323–329.

41 Barker, M.-J. (2013). Studying pornography. Available from: rewriting-the-rules.com/2013/06/01/studying-pornography.

42 Criminal Justice and Immigration Act (2008). Available from: legislation.gov.uk/ukpga/2008/4/section/63.

43 Ringrose, J., Gill, R., Livingstone, S., & Harvey, L. (2012). *A qualitative study of children, young people and 'sexting'*. NSPCC. Available from: eprints.lse.ac.uk/44216.

44 Stewart, R. S. (2019). Is feminist porn possible? *Sexuality & Culture, 23* (1), 254–270; O'Connor, R. (2013). What does feminist porn look like? *Everyday Feminism*. Available from: everydayfeminism.com/2013/09/feminist-porn.

45 Cardoso, D., & Paasonen, S. (2021). The value of print, the value of porn. *Porn Studies, 8* (1), 92–106; Fisher, W. A., & Barak, A. (1991). Pornography, erotica, and behavior: More questions than answers. *International Journal of Law and Psychiatry, 14* (1), 65–83.

46 Docz, E. (2015). One lawyer's crusade to defend extreme pornography. *The Guardian*. www.theguardian.com/law/2015/sep/09/one-lawyers-crusade-defend-extreme-pornography.

47 Backlash (2015). Origin story. Available from: www.backlash-uk.org.uk/origin-story-how-myles-jackman-became-obscenity-lawyer.

48 Bale, C. (2011). Raunch or romance? Framing and interpreting the relationship between sexualized culture and young people's sexual health. *Sex Education, 11* (3), 303–313.

49 Attwood, F., Smith, C., & Barker, M. (2021). Engaging with pornography: An examination of women aged 18–26 as porn consumers. *Feminist Media Studies, 21* (2), 173–188; Grubbs, J. B., Wright, P. J., Braden,

A. L., Wilt, J. A., & Kraus, S. W. (2019). Internet pornography use and sexual motivation: A systematic review and integration. *Annals of the International Communication Association*, 43 (2), 117–155.

50 Short, M. B., Black, L., Smith, A. H., Wetterneck, C. T., & Wells, D. E. (2012). A review of Internet pornography use research: Methodology and content from the past 10 years. *Cyberpsychology, Behavior, and Social Networking*, 15 (1), 13–23.

51 Antevska, A., & Gavey, N. (2015). 'Out of sight and out of mind' detachment and men's consumption of male sexual dominance and female submission in pornography. *Men and Masculinities*, 18 (5), 605–629.

52 Liberman, R. (2015). 'It's a really great tool': Feminist pornography and the promotion of sexual subjectivity. *Porn Studies*, 2 (2–3), 174–191.

53 McKee, A., Albury, K., Dunne, M., Grieshaber, S., Hartley, J., Lumby, C., & Mathews, B. (2010). Healthy sexual development: A multidisciplinary framework for research. *International Journal of Sexual Health*, 22 (1), 14–19.

54 McKee, A. (2010). Does pornography harm young people? *Australian Journal of Communication*, 37 (1), 17–36.

55 Goldfarb, E. S., & Lieberman, L. D. (2021). Three decades of research: The case for comprehensive sex education. *Journal of Adolescent Health*, 68 (1), 13–27.

56 Bragg, S., Ponsford, R., Meiksin, R., Emmerson, L., & Bonell, C. (2021). Dilemmas of school-based relationships and sexuality education for and about consent. *Sex Education*, 21 (3), 269–283; Renold, E. J., Ashton, M. R., & McGeeney, E. (2023). What if?: Becoming response-able with the making and mattering of a new relationships and sexuality education curriculum. In Kathryn J. Strom, Tammy Mills, Linda Abrams (Eds.), *Non-linear perspectives on teacher development* (pp. 342–359). Routledge.

57 Gauntlett, D. (2006). Ten things wrong with the media effects model. Available from: davidgauntlett.com/wp-content/uploads/2018/04/Ten-Things-Wrong-2006-version.pdf.

58 Heimer, K. (2019). Inequalities and crime. *Criminology*, 57 (3), 377–394.

59 Lombard, N. (2013). Violence against women starts with school stereotypes. *The Conversation*. Available from: theconversation.com/violence-against-women-starts-with-school-stereotypes-18440.

60 Everyday Sexism: everydaysexism.com.

61 Grogan, S. (2021). *Body image: Understanding body dissatisfaction in men, women and children*. Routledge.

62 Hust, S. J., Rodgers, K. B., Ebreo, S., & Stefani, W. (2019). Rape myth acceptance, efficacy, and heterosexual scripts in men's magazines: Factors associated with intentions to sexually coerce or intervene. *Journal of Interpersonal Violence*, 34 (8), 1703–1733.

63 Pozzulo, J. (2024). Rape myths can affect jurors' perceptions of sexual assault, and that needs to change. *The Conversation*. Available from: theconversation.com/rape-myths-can-affect-jurors-perceptions-of-sexual-assault-and-that-needs-to-change-235175.

64 Simic, Z. (2012). Why 'legitimate' rape and other myths are alive and dangerous. *The Conversation*. Available from: theconversation.com/why-legitimate-rape-and-other-myths-are-alive-and-dangerous-8988.

65 Reay, B., Attwood, N., & Gooder, C. (2013). Inventing sex: The short history of sex addiction. *Sexuality & Culture*, 17 (1), 1–19; Grubbs, J. B., Hoagland, K. C., Lee, B. N., Grant, J. T., Davison, P., Reid, R. C., & Kraus, S. W. (2020). Sexual addiction 25 years on: A systematic and methodological review of empirical literature and an agenda for future research. *Clinical Psychology Review*, 82, 101925.

66 Reid, R. C., & Kafka, M. P. (2014). Controversies about hypersexual disorder and the DSM-5. *Current Sexual Health Reports*, 6 (4), 259–264.

67 Joannides, P. (2012). The challenging landscape of problematic sexual behaviors, including 'sexual addiction' and 'hypersexuality'. In P. Kleinplatz (Ed.), *New directions in sex therapy: Innovations and alternatives* (pp. 69–83). Taylor & Francis.

68 COSRT (2021). *Common sexual problems*. Available from: cosrt.org.uk/wp-content/uploads/2021/08/Common-Sexual-Problems.pdf.

69 Davies, D., & Barker, M. J. (2015). Gender and sexuality diversity (GSD): Respecting difference. *The Psychotherapist*, 60, 16–17.

70 Ley, D. J. (2017). Sex addiction: An iatrogenic and moral concept. In Thaddeus Birchard, Joanna Benfield (Eds.), *Routledge international handbook of sexual addiction* (pp. 439–444). Routledge.

71 Irvine, J. M. (2014). Regulated passions: The invention of inhibited sexual desire and sex addiction. In Robert Granfield, Craig Reinarman (Eds.), *Expanding addiction: Critical essays* (pp. 233–248). Routledge.

72 Barker, M. (2013). Reflections: Towards a mindful sexual and relationship therapy. *Sexual Relationship Therapy*, 28 (1–2), 148–152.

73 For more on sexual compulsion, see: Neves, S. (2021). *Compulsive sexual behaviours: A psycho-sexual treatment guide for clinicians*. Routledge.

74 Barker, M. (2013). *Mindful counselling & psychotherapy: Practising mindfully across approaches and issues*. Sage.

75 I work through these ideas in depth, in relation to the gender wars, in: Barker, M. J., & Ryan-Flood, R. (2023). The gender wars and difficult conversations about trans: An interview with Meg-John Barker. In Róisín Ryan-Flood, Isabel Crowhurst, Laurie James-Hawkins (Eds.), *Difficult conversations* (pp. 11–26). Routledge.

6

UN/CONSCIOUS SEX

In previous chapters we touched on how psychoanalytic theories were one of the main building blocks for how we came to view sex as we currently do in psychology and more widely. We saw how Freud's ideas – about the aim and object of sex – shaped common understandings of people's sexuality being defined by the gender they're attracted to as well as what constitutes functional vs. dysfunctional, and normal vs. abnormal, sex. All this impacts the debates we have around sex, including which become objects of concern and how we approach them in polarised ways (as good/bad, right/wrong, etc.)

We might say that early psychoanalysis closed many things down in relation to how we understand and experience sex. Those who immediately followed Freud, in particular, rigidly delineated between supposedly healthy and unhealthy forms of sexual attraction, desire, and expression.[1] However, one vital thing that psychoanalysis opened up was a recognition of how much we humans are influenced by unconscious forces, not just in relation to our erotic lives but in all aspects of life.

In recent years, psychosocial theorists, relational therapists, trauma practitioners, intersectional feminists, and more have addressed how the traumatic experiences we have – within traumatising

DOI: 10.4324/9781003728979-6

societies – shape our erotic and intimate lives. That is what we'll turn to in this chapter. How do unconscious patterns play out through our sex lives? And how might we become more conscious about this, hopefully enabling more consensual, connected relating with ourselves, others, and the world?

Before we begin, just a reminder to go gently with yourself while reading this. All of us carry some form of cultural and personal trauma in relation to sex. There are ways of engaging with this, which we'll cover, which can bring us to a far more expansive and intimate relationship with ourselves and our sexualities. However, the process of acknowledging and addressing trauma is slow and often very painful in places. If trauma – particularly sexual trauma – is live for you at the moment, it's fine to leave this chapter for now. If you read on but find yourself feeling overwhelmed or confused at all, please do step away and look after yourself and consider accessing some support before coming back to it.[2]

UNCONSCIOUS SEX AND TRAUMA

Throughout this book we've explored how all of the following are hugely shaped by prevailing cultural understandings and by our personal experiences: what and who we find attractive and how we identify our sexualities (Chapter 2), the sex we do or don't engage in (Chapter 3), our sexual desires and what turns us on (Chapter 4), and our views and opinions about sex (Chapter 5).

All of this works through numerous complex biopsychosocial processes.[3] One simplified way of understanding these is that wider cultural meanings, and our own experiences over time, become laid down in our bodyminds[4] in ways we're not fully conscious of. These then manifest *through* us biopsychosocially, via our sensations, feelings, thoughts, words, and actions: a specific sight or smell brings up an erotic memory; being treated in a certain way leads to physical arousal; we find ourselves acting flirtatiously with someone we've just met or fiercely defending a certain opinion online.

In this section of the chapter we'll explore how what we might call our erotic unconscious is shaped by the following:

- *Sexual* cultures and personal experiences
- Specifically *traumatic* sexual cultures and personal experiences and
- Wider forms of cultural and personal trauma, which are not necessarily sexual

Our erotic unconscious

Perhaps the most obvious way our erotic unconscious is shaped by dominant culture and personal experience is where these explicitly relate to sex. This is what we've mostly focused on in the book so far.

For example, one way sexual cultures shape our unconscious is through explicit – and implicit – sex education. The *overt* sex ed curriculum often gives a clear impression of what constitutes sex, how we're expected to go about it, when, and who with. The *hidden* curriculum of what's not mentioned, as well as what forms of sexual behaviour are unquestioningly tolerated by the adults and peers around us, gives equally clear messages about what kinds of desires are unacceptable, what kinds of bodies are and aren't sexy, and who's allowed to do what to whom.[5]

Within such cultures, our own sexual experiences also shape our erotic unconscious. For example, if we learn how to give ourselves sexual pleasure early on this may enable us to be clearer with others about what kinds of stimulation our bodies like or to incorporate self touch into partnered sex. Alternatively – especially if others shame our early experiences of self-pleasure – it may lead to us separating off solo sex and partnered sex and struggling to derive pleasure from the latter. Whether our early sexual experiences take the form of mutual explorations, or of one or more people trying desperately to conform to a certain sexual script, will have a profound impact on where we go next erotically. We may well continue in this manner, or we may react against the form those early encounters took.[6]

Sexual trauma

It's important to be clear that not all of our unconscious learning, memories, and patterns relating to sex come from trauma. For example, we might access media representations and cultural stories about sexuality which enable us to find joy and pride in our identities or which open up sexual experiences that are highly pleasurable. Early experiences of excitement and contentment may become linked to certain situations or dynamics which serve us well in later life. For example, someone whose childhood delight is dressing up may find an enjoyable hobby or profession in burlesque or erotic dancing. Someone who finds a sense of freedom in being naked as a child may connect with communities later in life where people enjoy being naked together, in a sexual or non-sexual context.

However, traumatic cultural messages and personal experiences do have a profound influence on our erotic unconscious as well as on our unconscious more broadly. And this has a huge impact on how we experience our sexuality, our selves, and our relationships. That's why we'll focus on trauma for the remainder of the chapter.[7]

People are often cautious around the topic of trauma and sex, and for good reason. As we've seen, for many years Western psychology and dominant culture divided sexual attractions, identities, acts, and desires into:

- *Pathological* ones regarded as being shaped by trauma and requiring fixing or healing and
- *Non-pathological* ones regarded as normal and not requiring any intervention (see Chapter 4).

Recent authors such as Avgi Saketopoulou,[8] Ann Pellegrini,[9] and George Taxidis[10] challenge this division by taking what they call a 'traumatophilic' approach to sex. They regard all of our sexualities as being shaped by trauma. Therefore, it's just as valuable for those who're sexually normative to address their trauma as it is for those who are sexually non-normative. While never trivialising the often devastating impacts of trauma, they invite everyone to get curious about its workings and how they might engage with it in themselves, rather than trying to eradicate it or fix it entirely.

This is the kind of approach I'm following here. Those who fit within the current sexual norms, those who fall outside of them, and those – many more – who *appear* normative but actually have non-normative desires, attractions, or experiences are *all* impacted by traumatising cultures and experiences. And all of us may benefit from becoming more conscious and curious about our sexualities and about ourselves more broadly.

This book has already covered how culturally traumatising ways of understanding sex restrict and constrain our sexualities. Within societies that delineate good and bad kinds of sex, many people will embrace and express desires and attractions which fit the 'good' category and repress or disown any which fit the 'bad'. Those of us who question such cultural norms – or who can't force our bodyminds to conform to them – may well internalise shame around our marginalised sexualities. For those who do conform, the disowned and repressed elements may leak – or lash – out unexpectedly at times: Gayle Rubin's 'something unspeakable' may 'skitter across'.[11] It can be very frightening, shaming – and potentially harmful to ourselves and others – when we act out of unconscious cravings and aversions.

Turning to personal experience, research on sexual trauma highlights the profound and damaging impact it generally has on survivors' lives and on their mental health.[12] The focus is often on what's called 'big T' trauma, in the form of violent sexual assault or childhood sexual abuse. However, it's important to emphasise that trauma – sexual and otherwise – takes many forms. For example, the cumulative impact of more minor seeming incidents can be just as impactful as one major one. Also, the way people around the survivor respond is pivotal in how the trauma impacts them. For example, those who don't feel safe enough to share what's happened – or who are met with a dismissive, minimising, or victim-blaming response – will likely be far more damaged by the experience than those who are taken seriously and supported by those around them.[13]

Sexual trauma has distressing impacts on our erotic lives specifically. It can leave us unable to enjoy our eroticism at all or in particular ways. It can leave us experiencing arousal in places linked to the trauma, which can be deeply distressing and confusing.

Of course, we can't completely disentangle cultural and personal forms of trauma as traumatising cultures are a major reason why interpersonal trauma happens. For example, denial and victim blaming are key features of rape culture,[14] which is a major reason why people often respond to survivors in minimising and judgemental ways, including in mental health services and criminal justice systems.[15] In her classic book on trauma, Judith Herman outlines how – in psychology and in dominant culture – each time there's been a wave of increased awareness of just how many children and adults experience sexual trauma, this has been followed by a backlash wave of denial.[16] For example, Freud backtracked on his early work, which documented the extent of sexual abuse and assault he witnessed among his clients, after this was derided by his colleagues. When second-wave feminism demonstrated just how many women and children were being sexually abused and assaulted in the home, this was followed by a moral panic around false memories. It's important that we don't use research findings about the eroticisation of trauma, or the way memories are constructed over time, to downplay or deny the extent or impact of sexual trauma.[17]

Another link between cultural and personal trauma is the fact we pass on traumatising ways of doing sex and relationships through intergenerational trauma. For example, in communities where there's a lot of anxiety and shame about sex, these messages get passed on in families, schools, and so on, both through what's said and through what's not said. This leads to confusion, misinformation, and internal anxiety and shame, which shapes our personal experiences. For example, we may have no sense that it's okay not to be sexual. We may be unable to allow non-normative or stigmatised sexual attractions or desires in ourselves or others. Or we may have little sense of how to go about sex with another person in a way that's consensual because we've never witnessed people relating in such ways.

Cultural and personal trauma and sex

In the previous sections, we've considered the ways *sexual* cultures and *sexual* experiences shape us, particularly traumatising sexual cultures and experiences. However, the impact of wider culture and personal experience on sex goes far beyond this.

Cultural trauma

Beginning with culture, being embedded in dominant forms of colonial and capitalist culture[18] has a profound – while often invisible – impact on how we relate to ourselves and others, including erotically.

For example, key features of such cultures include the following:[19]

- Individuals, communities, and nations regard areas of land as their property, displacing or eliminating any humans and other living organisms currently occupying it, extracting resources from it, and – often violently – forbidding others access to it and protecting its borders against potential attack.
- Humans, and other beings, are divided into those regarded as less or more valid and valuable, with the enslavement or exploitation of those deemed less so on behalf of those deemed more so, including treating the former as disposable, and less worthy of a liveable life.
- Individuals, communities, and nations are regarded as separate from each other and in competition with each other for scarce resources. Their ways of knowing and being are pitched in opposition to one another, with 'us' needing to be proved and defended as right, good, and superior compared to 'them', who must be wrong, bad, and inferior.

- There's a constant seeking for 'us' and 'our people' to obtain *more* of everything including success, happiness, wealth, and power and to avoid pain, suffering, and death.

It may seem a stretch to link industrial fishing trawlers destroying the ocean ecosystem and forcing local fishing communities to starve or leave their homes to our personal erotic lives, but really it's not.[20] Cultural trauma impacts sex *directly*, for example, in how sexual violence gets used as a weapon in warfare or how the isolation of pandemic lockdowns deprive people of touch. Cultural trauma also impacts sex *indirectly*, via unconscious processes. For example, taking the features of colonialism and capitalism listed above, we might consider how common it is to believe the following:

- Sexual partners should consistently feel certain ways about us. Their bodies should continue to look a certain way over time and respond to us in certain ways in order to demonstrate our desirability. Partners should share our desires and opinions. Whether or not we treat them well, and whether our relationship continues, is contingent on this. This could be seen as a kind of colonising of partners' bodies, minds, and feelings (and our own, when we try to force ourselves to continue feeling and responding in certain ways).
- There's a scale of sexual attractiveness with those higher up being more valuable than those lower down. We must force our bodies, minds, and characters to meet these standards because it entitles us to certain kinds of sex and respect.[21]
- We need to compete with others to obtain sexual partners and prove and defend our worthiness – to others and ourselves – on the basis of how many partners we've had, how good we are at sex, how exciting our sex life is, how well we treat others sexually, or other measures of sexual prowess.
- There's a goal to sex and we need to push ourselves and others to reach this, whether that be penetration, orgasm, a transcendent state, or affirmation of loving connection (see Chapter 3).

> Sex which doesn't meet our needs is a problem, and all 'negative' feelings, sensations, and experiences must be kept out of sex.[22]

We might regard colonial and capitalist cultures as traumatised and traumatising. This is not just because of their destructive impact on humans, other beings, and the planet but also because of their impact on our unconscious mindsets and how these harm us and others through our words and actions, including sexual ones. When we're embedded in such cultures – and have been all our lives – it can be painful indeed to recognise how they operate through us, and long, slow work to reckon with this and to find other ways of being and relating.[23]

Within such cultures, there's a risk that those who *do* become aware of these things will tragically use the same kind of traumatising approach to *address* it in themselves and others. For example, we may beat ourselves up for behaving in the ways described with partners past or present. We may become invested in the view of ourselves and our communities as the 'good', 'pure' ones who see the right of things, repressing and disowning our own 'bad', 'impure' thoughts and feelings, projecting those out onto others and policing and punishing them out there.[24] It's helpful to keep in mind Audre Lorde's famous quote: 'the master's tools will never dismantle the master's house'.[25] Or, as Báyò Akómoláfé puts it: 'just because we are tirelessly against something doesn't mean we are excused from its operational logic'.[26] We'll return, towards the end of the chapter, to how we might shift sexual cultures over time and how this could be part of a wider cultural transformation.

Personal trauma

Turning to personal experience, a burgeoning body of work in recent decades suggests that we're profoundly shaped by developmental trauma. This happens in our early relationships and is often replicated and reinforced in our later relationships as well.

Again, developmental trauma is interwoven with cultural trauma rather than separate from it.[27] For example, historical forms of trauma experienced collectively by a community are often passed on directly and indirectly through the generations.[28] Also, traumatising cultures often mean that adults aren't able to parent in ways that would enable children to grow up less traumatised. They may be too stretched due to working under conditions of poverty or austerity. There may be few state or community resources for people parenting in nuclear or single-parent family contexts. They may not have had the opportunity, encouragement, or support to acknowledge and address their own trauma.

Developmental trauma occurs when children experience feelings which are too overwhelming for them to process alone and which aren't 'held and heard' by anybody else in their lives.[29] This means they don't gradually learn how to contain such feelings themselves or that it's okay to have them and to share them with others. As mentioned before, such overwhelming feelings can be the result of 'big T' traumas such as having a bad accident or experiencing abuse or neglect. However, they can also be the result of cumulative experiences which may not be culturally recognised as trauma but can have just as a huge impact on a developing child. Additionally, because these things can happen so early in life, we may never know some of their origins for sure.

The combination of the overwhelming experience *and* whether or not it's held and heard by anyone else is crucial. For example, imagine a child who experiences inappropriate sexual touch or comments from a peer or family member. Things will be very different for them if people in their life notice that something is wrong, encourage them to talk about it and feel its impact, and do something about the situation than it will if there's a collusion of silence and the experience is denied, belittled, or blamed on the child themselves. Sadly such responses are all too common.

Trauma researchers suggest that when trauma isn't processed at the time it becomes locked in our bodyminds.[30] We develop stories about – and patterns of relating with – ourselves and others, as well as ways of holding our bodies, to avoid the overwhelming, unbearable feelings which remain hidden away.[31] In the next section we'll turn to these kinds of stories and patterns and how they can show up in sex. After this we'll address how we can become more conscious about trauma and address it in our erotic lives.

TRAUMA AND CONSENT

When we carry unprocessed trauma in our bodyminds, it can be triggered by things that happen in the present. We can, at such times, find ourselves reliving past trauma in the form of flashbacks. This is when we're flooded by emotions like shame, rage, terror, or longing which feel overwhelming and unbearable. We may find ourselves unable to prevent memories from replaying or thought processes from spiralling. Our bodies may brace, flinch, or clench. Words and actions may play out, seemingly beyond our control, as if what happened before is happening right now. When trauma happened early, cumulatively over time, and/or in ways we were forbidden from acknowledging in our family or community, such experiences can be horribly confusing. It can be unclear what triggered them or why they're happening.[32]

For many people, much of the time, trauma isn't experienced this vividly because we've developed unconscious strategies which protect us from feeling that level of pain. Even when triggered, we may not experience the unbearable feelings directly but go straight to one of these protective survival strategies. Over time such strategies can become deeply entrenched patterns of understanding – and relating with – ourselves, others, and the world. Our whole character may become fixed around one particular strategy, or we may oscillate between them, with different ones becoming our go-to in particular situations or dynamics. These survival strategies often become so familiar to us – and to those around us – that we don't even see them *as* strategies, they're just us. Some of them are normalised in cultures where so many of us are traumatised in particular ways.

Survival strategies

There are many ways of naming and describing the common survival strategies, and we may react in complex combinations of these ways as well as in different ways at different times. However, a simple model can be useful for orienting ourselves. Figure 6.1 combines and adapts two approaches which I find particularly helpful:[33]

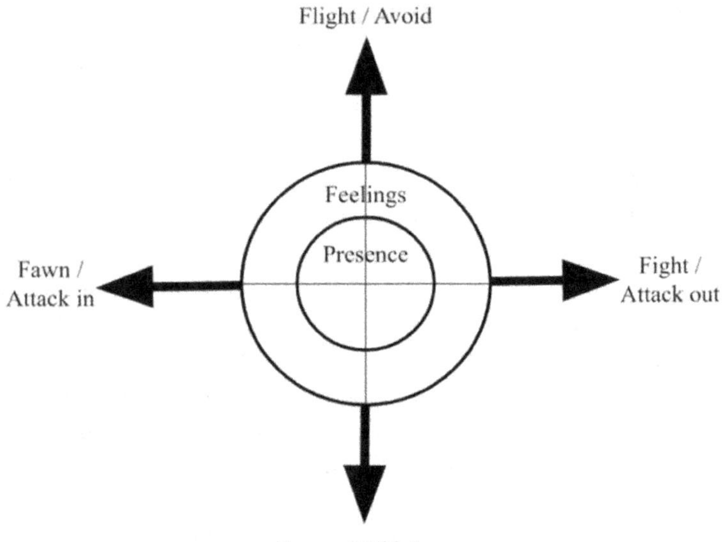

FIGURE 6.1 Trauma compass

If we imagine the overwhelming unprocessed feelings around us in the centre of the compass, then the compass points are the strategies we go to in order to avoid feeling them.

These strategies are all versions of the ways organisms naturally respond to immediate threat in order to survive: fleeing, fighting, freezing, or fawning to appease a threatening other. However, such strategies become ingrained habits of protecting ourselves, often from situations which are now psychologically – rather than existentially – dangerous (e.g. threats to how we see ourselves or how others see us, rather than threats to our life or freedom). This may be because, when we were very young, psychological risk *was* also dangerous to our life. If a caregiver rejected us we literally wouldn't survive.

Here's a brief summary of how these four survival strategies work:

- In *flight*, or avoid, we tend to repress painful feelings or dissociate from them, often by keeping ourselves busy or distracted and by performing a kind of 'good' self in the world.
- In *fight*, or attack out, we tend to believe that others – or external circumstances – are responsible for our painful feelings. We judge and criticise them or try to control them to make them better, so the feelings will go away.
- In *freeze*, or withdraw, we try to escape anything which might trigger our painful feelings, often restricting our engagement with others and the world in various ways.
- In *fawn*, or attack in, we tend to believe we, ourselves, are responsible for our painful feelings, and we attempt to shape ourselves in ways others will approve of, believing this will protect us from the feelings.

Over the course of our lives, as we relate to challenging situations from these survival strategies rather than feeling the emotions they bring up, the amount of pain we haven't processed accumulates. This can make it even harder to turn and face it, and therefore, more likely we'll employ our survival strategies, creating a vicious circle. The resistance required in the survival strategies to hold back *that* much pain can become a major kind of suffering itself.

Trauma, survival strategies, and sex

All of this can play out in relation to sex. In fact, it might be particularly likely in this area, given how sex often involves being vulnerable and exposed, surrendering or letting go in ways which leave us open to deep feelings surfacing. Also, given how interwoven love, sex, and partnership are in dominant culture, sexual relationships are often the ones we – unconsciously – look to to address earlier relational trauma. This means they're also frequently the relationships most likely to trigger overwhelming feelings when similar things seem to be playing out there as happened to us as before.

For example, if we're someone who repeatedly had our boundaries overstepped as a child – whether sexually or non-sexually – we may well be triggered in the present if somebody touches us in ways we haven't agreed to, whether that's in everyday life or in a sexual context. Such experiences may bring up unbearable feelings for us, and perhaps also confusing memories, or imaginings of sexual violence. Depending on the patterns we've developed, we may find ourselves pushing those feelings down or trying to distract from them (*flight*). We may attack whoever has overstepped our boundaries, while perhaps finding it very hard to determine whether it was deliberate or not or how big a violation it was (*fight*). We might go numb and allow whatever is happening or fearfully try to ensure that we never encounter that person again (*freeze*). We might tell ourselves it was our fault this happened or even try to convince ourselves – and the other person – that it was something we wanted (*fawn*).

If we're someone who hasn't received enough affection or touch as a child, in a situation with someone we feel drawn to we may find unbearable feelings start to swirl. Depending on our patterns – and the situation – we may shove those feelings down and relate with that person in a superficial way (*flight*). We may feel angry with that person, perceiving them as denying us something we're entitled to (*fight*). Perhaps we'll *freeze* whenever we're around them, finding ourselves dissociated or struggling to speak. Or maybe we'll hungrily latch onto this person, obsessing about them, or even crossing their boundaries in an attempt to get close to them (*fawn*).

As you can imagine from these examples, when people with different kinds of trauma – or different survival strategies – relate, it's very easy for them to get into cycles of repeatedly triggering each other.

Such strategies can become our go-to ways of relating with sex in general. For example, someone who tends towards *flight* may use sex as one of their ways of staying busy and distracted, such as spending a lot of time on apps or dating. Alternatively, they may be more likely to engage in sex in quite a disconnected way, going through the motions or performing rather than being present. Someone who tends towards *fight* may exert power and dominance in sexual ways, viewing it as a conquest. Or they may try to control sex in order to get what they want out of it. Someone who tends towards *freeze* may disengage from sex or be very cautious about the kinds of sex they engage with. Or they may engage a lot with particular kinds of sex they find safe or soothing. Someone who tends towards *fawn* may have quite a craving approach to sex, seeking it out to get the feelings of connection or approval they yearn for. Or they may engage in unwanted sex in order to please a partner, pretending to enjoy it. Of course, these are just a few possibilities, and there are many other ways such strategies can play out.[34]

When it comes to intimate relationships more broadly, we might see survival strategies show up, for example, in avoiding deeper intimacies or keeping people at bay (*flight*), in attempting to control partners and make them into what we want (*fight*), in physically or emotionally withdrawing in moments of tension or heightened emotion (*freeze*), or in continually seeking intense connection with the same person or different people (*fawn*). Trauma can mean we're drawn to relationships which operate in the kinds of abusive or neglectful ways that are familiar from our early relationships, keeping us stuck in painful cycles.

Trauma, survival strategies, and consent

When we're triggered into unprocessed trauma and overwhelming feelings and when we're operating out of unconscious survival strategies, it becomes much more difficult – even impossible – to treat ourselves and others consensually. When we don't have much awareness of trauma and how it operates – or much support to address our own trauma – we may not realise this is what's happening: it may feel so familiar or normal to us. This is compounded by the fact that being treated in some way non-consensually by others, or by wider culture, is such a common type of traumatising experience.

When we're triggered into a flashback, we may perceive those around us as the ones who were involved in our past trauma and find ourselves speaking and acting towards them as if they were. Our body may shake or flail and we may have little control over our speech or actions. The degree of danger or desperation we feel may mean we act in ways which are non-consensual towards ourselves or others. For example, we may find it impossible to seek support, we may try to escape our distress in ways which hurt us, or we may seek support from others in ways which require more of them than they can offer.

Similarly, when we're stuck in a survival strategy in order not to feel those overwhelming unprocessed emotions, we can often struggle to treat ourselves and others consensually. In *flight* we may be too distant from our bodies and feelings to tune into what we want or don't want or to pick up on others' discomfort. In *fight* others may get the sense we'll attack them if they don't go along with what we want or if we feel rejected by them saying 'no' to something. We may have so much suspicion and distrust of others that it's impossible for us to relax in the way we'd need in order to be in self-consent. In *freeze* we may be too frightened or dissociated to tune into potentially pleasurable things or to be honest with others about how we're doing. In *fawn* we might be so focused on the other person's desires, or ensuring they aren't disappointed in us, that we struggle to know what we'd like. Others may feel objectified by our focus on them or pressured to go along with something by our need for their approval.

Understandably, many of us would like simple, straightforward guidelines to ensure that sex – and everything – is consensual. It can be tempting to assume that people are all rational agents who always know whether or not they want to do things and can easily express their 'yes', 'no', or 'maybe' to others. However, personal trauma – and the unconscious patterns that result from it – actually make it very difficult indeed to tune into our desires and extremely hard to feel safe enough to convey these to another person. Add to this all the cultural pressures there are to be a certain kind of self who expresses their sexuality in a certain kind of way, and consent becomes massively challenging.

This is one reason why the kinds of consent cultures we covered in Chapter 4 are so vital and why such cultures also need to be trauma-informed: supporting and resourcing people to address their trauma. This is something we'll return to in the final section of the chapter, when we explore how we might become more conscious about how we treat ourselves and others, erotically and beyond.

Before that, let's consider how our sexuality itself can be a way into better understanding ourselves, the trauma we carry, and the survival strategies we act out of.

THE EROTIC IMAGINATION

When our strategies – and the cultural and personal traumas which led to them – operate unconsciously, it can be hard to identify them or to be aware of how they manifest in our lives. This is one reason why therapists have paid so much attention to dreams and to dynamics which play out between therapist and client. These can illuminate what may have happened in the past and the survival strategies we employ now.

The themes and dynamics that play out in our erotic imagination can be similarly revealing. This means they're a valuable resource when it comes to understanding ourselves better, and becoming more conscious in how we relate, erotically and otherwise.

Fantasies may take the form of verbal or visual stories we tell ourselves in our minds or images or words that pop up. If we don't actively engage in fantasy, we can tune into the erotic imagination by noticing the porn, erotica, or romance fiction we're drawn to or the scenes in mainstream media we're aroused by. We can observe the kinds of erotic roles, dynamics, and activities we like to act out online or offline.

Before we go on, think about whether you have recurring sexual fantasies or imaginings. What are your favourite ones? You might find it useful to write them down so you can think about them in relation to the ideas we'll explore here.[35]

Trauma and fantasy

As we saw in Chapter 4, many of the sexual desires which have been labelled 'abnormal' are actually very common. For example, Justin Lehmiller[36] found that nearly 90% of people fantasised about having a threesome, around two thirds some form of BDSM, and a similar number some form of open relationships. A large proportion fantasised about sex in unusual places or with somebody other than their partner. Also common was fantasising about deeply meaningful sex and being found highly desirable. Over half of straight women and nearly a third of straight men said they had fantasies about sex with people of the same gender. Popular collections of erotic fantasies generally include similar themes to these, helpfully normalising such desires for those who've been troubled by them.[37]

Trauma practitioners often link trauma to having been restricted in some way – culturally and/or personally – in relation to our freedom, our dignity, our safety, or our belonging.[38] A big part of collective and developmental trauma is having to make painful – often unconscious – choices to sacrifice one or more of these things in order to get the others. For example, if we find ourselves living in a community where our values aren't respected, we may sacrifice our freedom and dignity in order to belong there in relative safety. If the people around us during childhood were unsafe, we might later sacrifice any hope of finding belonging, prioritising freedom and dignity in order to avoid such treatment again. Many people hold trauma around the restriction of freedom, dignity, safety, and/or belonging. This often manifests in feelings of shame, rage, terror, or longing around being trapped, abandoned, annihilated, or rejected.

Many of the most common fantasies listed above reflect these themes of freedom, dignity, safety, and belonging. They imagine a world where, for example, we're free to express our sexuality wherever – and with whoever – we want, without being attacked or rejected, even being actively welcomed or desired for doing so. They play with themes of being trapped, betrayed, attacked, or humiliated. Common fantasies often draw on real-world forms of cultural trauma where freedom, dignity, safety, or belonging are restricted, including abduction and imprisonment, dominance and abuse of power, torture and punishment, servitude and enslavement.[39] Fantasies either render these experiences themselves hot or tell a story in which they culminate in our being freed, desired, rescued, or welcomed.

Exploring our fantasies

Some psychotherapists have conducted in-depth analyses of fantasies to explore what we can learn about ourselves by tuning into them. In the 1990s, US humanistic therapist Jack Morin wrote *The Erotic Mind*, based on his 'sexual excitement survey' with hundreds of people, as well as detailed analysis of the specific sexual fantasies of many of his clients.[40] In the 2000s, UK psychoanalyst Brett Kahr conducted an even more extensive survey of nearly 20,000 people and over a hundred in-depth interviews about people's lives and fantasies. This research formed the basis of his book *Sex and The Psyche*.[41] These authors agree that our recurring fantasies are often rooted in early trauma and have much to tell us about the fears and longings, cravings and aversions that stem from that.

Morin proposes an erotic equation: Excitement = Attraction + Obstacles. In other words, we tend to find it arousing when we're attracted to something and there's some difficulty to be overcome in order to get it. For example, a common theme in erotic fan fiction is the 'first time' story, where it isn't clear whether a character's attraction is reciprocated, but it turns out that it is when they're finally brave enough to confess. Also common are 'hurt comfort' stories, where a person has to endure some pain to get to the pleasure. There are also common themes of people having taboo desires (same-sex attraction or BDSM, for example) which are then fulfilled.[42] Morin's equation perhaps explains why so many common fantasies are about things which are socially taboo and why partially clothed can be sexier than completely naked! It also relates back to Esther Perel's work about the difficulties of maintaining passion in long-term relationships (see Chapter 3). Perhaps warm, close relationships don't provide us with enough sense of an obstacle to be hot.[43] Paradoxically Morin finds the things that can get in the way of desire – like guilt, anger, fear, and loneliness – can also amplify it, in small doses.

For Morin and Kahn this gives a clue to where our core erotic themes come from. While we're rarely conscious of it, we seem to use sexual fantasies to transform the obstacles of traumatic experiences from our past into excitement and pleasure. Both authors give powerful examples where a client describes a compelling fantasy which makes no sense to them, but probing into their past makes it crystal clear. For example, a person who experienced lots of unrequited love might fantasise about being in the midst of an orgy, utterly desired by all, or whisked away by a romantic hero. Someone who was bullied and rejected at school might turn the tables and be the dominant one in their fantasies, or they might imagine similar scenarios to the bullying but where it's consensual and pleasurable for them to submit. A person who was shamed for their bodily functions in the past may imagine pissing on other people or being carefully washed clean after such a thing happened to them.

As you can see, traumatic experiences seem to lodge in the erotic minds of different people in different manners, and fantasies operate in uniquely personal ways to address them.

Our plural selves

As well as exploring the themes and dynamics in our fantasies from a trauma perspective, it can be useful to explore the characters who show up there. Many therapists see all the beings who populate our dreams as representing aspects of ourselves. We can apply that theory to our daydreams and fantasies too.

Such an approach connects with many psychologies which see our selves as plural rather than singular. This is the idea that we're composed of a whole system or community, rather than each of us being a coherent individual unit.[44] There are many different understandings and experiences of plurality,[45] whether it's a vivid sense of being more than one self or a more muted awareness of having an inner child or inner critic, for example, or acting quite differently across different relationships or situations.[46] Approaches which link well with what we've covered in this chapter see the four compass points that we covered earlier as selves, parts, or subpersonalities.

For example, the psychoanalyst Ronald Fairburn suggested we all develop a performing self who acts in the world in ways we've been taught will be accepted and approved of. We push down into the unconscious a needy self who holds all the trauma of *losing* connection with others and is highly invested in getting it back. And we push down a rejected self who holds all the trauma of *being* disconnected from others and is invested in punishing others for this or trying to reform them into who we wish they would be.[47] These three selves map well onto the **flight**, *fawn*, and **fight** compass positions we covered earlier.

Relationship writers Jessica Fern and David Cooley map out three similar selves in their work: rescuer, shame, and critic.[48] They describe how these selves' strategies play out internally in relation to each other, for example, in the form of desperate inner children or brutal inner critics making demands on the performing self. Returning to our previous reflections on freedom, dignity, safety, and belonging, we might say that the performing self tries to repress the others in order to *freely* function in the world, while – unconsciously – the needy self pulls us towards **belonging**, the rejected self **dignity**, and a further – withdrawing – self prioritises *safety* over the risks of trying to belong or assert our freedom.

Some people may have certain selves as more of their go-to, with their overall character shaped particularly around being accomplished, truth-telling, timid, or 'keeping people sweet', for example. However, we all have all of these selves, and they often play out more or less in different situations and relationships in our lives. Frequently more than one self will be triggered simultaneously by the events of our life, kicking in with their stories and strategies. This can be very confusing as we find ourselves in internal conflict over whether we or someone else is to blame, for example, or torn between choices which seemingly offer more potential for freedom, dignity, safety, or belonging. Plural selves also internalise the cultural and community norms around us, using those to attack others – and us – for certain kinds of behaviour, for example, or to pull us towards certain kinds of relationships they believe will meet their needs or shame us for not having them.

Tragically the strategies of each self can leave them – and us – with the very opposite of what they long for: performing selves end up trapped in their performance, rejecting selves leave us disrespected by others because of how they criticise and blame, withdrawing selves find less and less safety as they make our worlds smaller and smaller, and needy selves push people away or get embroiled in painful relationships marked by loss of connection.

Our erotic selves

Attending to our erotic imaginations can help us to see how these four – and other – selves show up in us, what trauma stories they (and we) particularly carry, and what they may need in order to loosen their survival strategies. When we attend to the characters in our fantasies and the kinds of things they eroticise, we may find one self in each of these positions, or we may find whole systems of selves with different functions, or selves who sit between the different compass points.

For example, performing selves may fantasise about being trapped in being a certain way for others, about being exposed, or about rescuing others (*flight*). Rejecting selves may have dominant/sadistic fantasies of being desired and powerful, punishing or training others, or fantasies relating to the ways they were abused or betrayed (*fight*). Withdrawing selves may fantasise about being rescued or being safe and contained alone (*freeze*). Needy selves may have submissive/masochistic fantasies about being abject and desperate, about being punished or trained, or about belonging to someone or everyone (*fawn*).

Returning to the trauma compass, tuning into erotic fantasies might help us to describe in more detail how these selves – or self systems – work in us, for example (Figure 6.2):

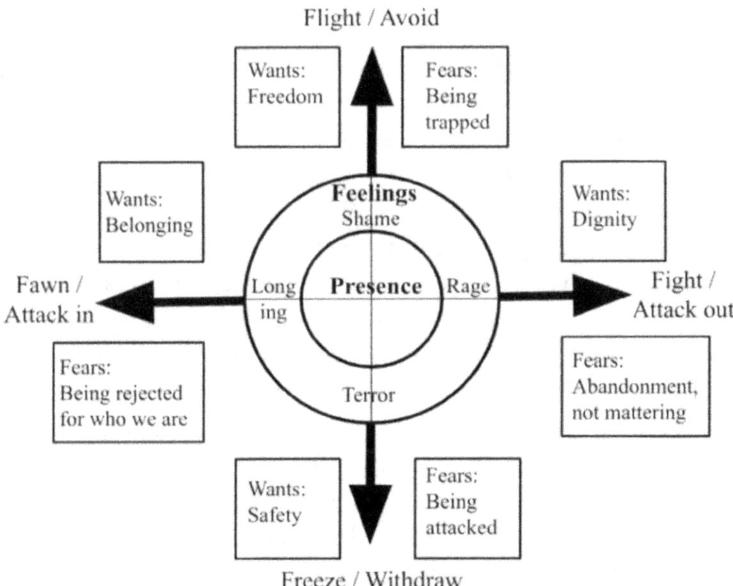

FIGURE 6.2 Expanded trauma compass

It's possible to creatively engage with our fantasies to excavate or cultivate selves, such as wise, caring, or parental selves or wild free selves who represent what we might have been like had we not experienced trauma. We can also use our erotic imagination to nurture relationships between all these selves, so that the 'inner children' who carry our earlier pain can finally be held and heard and get what they need (which may be different to what they seem to want!) as well as coming into more loving relationship with all the other selves. In this way what has been unconscious can become more conscious.

If we're to be able to do this kind of deep work with our erotic imaginations, we need shame-sensitive, trauma-informed approaches towards our fantasies and desires and towards forms of solo sex.[49] We need cultures which understand that – due to the nature of trauma – we may well eroticise forms of cultural and developmental trauma, including those relating to abuses of power and early childhood.

In their work on fantasies, Blake explores how we can be caring and consensual with ourselves and others when our fantasies relate to personal or collective histories of trauma.[50] While playing with such material – and selves – can be deeply fulfilling, arousing, and informative, doing so without carefully constructed containers, or a good understanding of the operation of trauma, can lead to us retraumatising ourselves or others. This is particularly the case if we're not aware of where these things are coming from, if we're scared to acknowledge them, or if we fixate on a particular person – or kind of sex – as the only place we can explore and embody them. The sense that we are – in a very real way – relating to wounded children within us, stuck at the time the trauma occurred, can be a helpful reminder of how careful we need to be.

Another risk is that we might keep these things purely in the realm of sex – seeing our plural selves as 'just' role plays or fantasy figures – rather than listening to what they're telling us about our unconscious stories and strategies and addressing these.

We'll turn now to the kinds of practices and supports which may be helpful with this.

CONSCIOUS SEX

Once we have a sense of how trauma can play out through sex and how intertwined our erotic desires often are with cultural and personal trauma, we're left with the question of how we might become more conscious about sex (and everything). Given that our trauma triggers and unconscious survival strategies make it difficult to treat ourselves – and others – consensually, becoming more personally – and collectively–- conscious is a vital part of cultivating consent cultures (see Chapter 4).

The intention of *conscious* sex is to nurture our capacity to be present during sex of all kinds and tuned in to how we and others are doing. It also involves noticing when we've gone *unconscious* in any way: triggered into overwhelming feelings or survival strategies. It enables us to articulate to ourselves and others when that has happened to stop or pause and bring ourselves back – accessing support to do this if necessary.

Addressing (sexual) trauma

When we carry unprocessed trauma and our survival strategies are deeply embedded, such conscious sex may feel a long way off. Thankfully there are now many ways of addressing trauma, including sexual trauma. It's perfectly fine to take a break from sex while we do the work of addressing our trauma or to only engage in certain forms of sex which feel safe enough during such times.

Most approaches to trauma have in common that they enable us to finally feel the feelings we were trying to avoid with our survival patterns in a way that doesn't overwhelm us. In this way we can finally hold and hear the parts of us – or places within us – which carry the trauma. We can finally process what happened in the past, allowing us to loosen the restrictive stories and strategies which continue to hurt us – and others – in the present.

Here are some examples of therapies and practices which can help us to do this work:

- Many forms of meditation and mindfulness help us develop the capacity to slow down, to refrain from acting out of our survival strategies, and to feel the feelings under our storylines or thought processes.[51] If these are trauma-informed they will stress going slowly, accessing the support of teachings and community, and building routines and rituals to scaffold our practice.[52]

- Somatic therapies and practices emphasise that trauma is locked in our bodies so embodied techniques can be particularly helpful in addressing it. This can include attending to parts of our body in certain ways, physical movement of some kind, or therapies and guided practices which include touch.[53] Somatic sexologists and sexological bodyworkers can work directly with sexuality in embodied ways.[54]
- Trauma-informed therapists, counsellors, and coaches emphasise that most of our trauma occurs in relational contexts, so it can be hugely valuable to address it in relationship. A trauma-informed therapist can hold and hear our trauma, helping us to increase our capacity to hold and hear it ourselves. They can also help us to understand how our survival strategies play out with others, in a safe-enough container where the other person hopefully won't go into *their* survival strategies in response and where we can practise alternative ways of relating with others.[55] If we're particularly focused on sexual trauma or how trauma shows up in sex, then a sex therapist, or practitioner trained on gender, sex, and relationship diversity, might be most helpful.[56] Many trauma practitioners work with plural parts or selves.[57]
- Given that so much of our trauma is collective – a result of growing up in traumatised and traumatising cultures – it can be helpful to address it in community. Supportive groups offer a collective space for engaging with trauma. This can include the holding and hearing of trauma by the group, often by those who have been through similar things themselves. Groups are also spaces where we can practise new ways of relating with others and be supported by particular structures and rituals.[58] We may find such support through specific sexual communities, such as feminist, survivor, or LGBTQIA+ movements.
- Given the disconnection with land common to many capitalist and colonialist cultures, people often find re/connecting with

nature to be helpful when addressing trauma. We can feel held and heard in wide open spaces or by ancient trees or bodies or water, and we can learn different ways of relating with plants, animals, or weather. Some therapies explicitly engage people with nature and the more-than-human world to provide structures and support for this.[59] Many people also find support with this kind of work through their faith or spiritual communities and practices.

This might feel like a bewildering array of options. It's important to remember that different things work for different people and at different points in their lives. Explore the ones which feel like the best fit for where you're at. Similarly, the fit between you and any practitioner or community is vital. It's important to shop around and find ones which feel affordable and safe enough for you, avoiding any individuals or communities who suggest they know better than you know yourself or who feel at all rushed or pushy. One thing all trauma approaches agree on is how essential it is to go slowly.

Conscious engagement with what is unconscious runs counter to mainstream culture, and indeed to many psychologies, given how focused these often are on fixing what's 'wrong' with people so they can go back to 'normal' functioning and productivity as quickly as possible. Returning to that notion of 'traumatophilic' practice, this work is not about eradicating distressing feelings, resolving the past, and following a linear path to complete healing or recovery. Rather it's a slow, gradual, spiralling process through which we become increasingly able to encompass our overwhelming feelings, to be with our painful memories, to love our traumatised selves, and to expand from stuck patterns into other possibilities.[60]

Mindful sex

An activity I've often done in workshops about sex is to encourage everyone to think of a particular erotic or sensual activity they engage with, such as sharing a kiss, getting a massage, fantasising, masturbating, or having a particular kind of sex with a partner. Once they've picked an activity, participants try to remember a time when they found that activity really fulfilling and another time when it was unfulfilling (nothing non-consensual or traumatic, just not particularly enjoyable or satisfying).

You might like to try this for yourself before moving on. You can write a brief description – a paragraph or so – of the fulfilling version and the unfulfilling version. Then reflect on what the main differences were between the two versions.

Whether workshop attendees were therapists, students, or kinksters, and whatever activities they focused on, the differences people noticed were very similar. Broadly speaking, in fulfilling versions of the activity, people felt more:

- Present to what was happening and less distracted
- Embodied and tuned in to their sensations and feelings
- Open and curious as to what might unfold, flexible, and flowing rather than trying to reach any particular goal or outcome
- Connected with themselves and with anybody else involved
- Able to be vulnerable and kind towards themselves and with anybody else involved

You might remember that many of these points are emphasised in the kind of sex therapy we explored towards the end of Chapter 3. This focuses not on *what* kind of sex people have – and trying to enable this – but rather on *how* we engage with our eroticism: enabling people to shift towards something more like what's described in this list.

The features listed here are also a pretty good description of how we can be – more broadly – in our lives when we're not triggered into flashbacks or engaged in survival strategies. Many of us, sadly, may only know this way of being through glimpses and glimmers, for example, when struck by a beautiful sight outdoors, while dancing or swimming, during the early phases of a new relationship or in a crowd watching a powerful concert or sporting event.

Being mindful – or just being – describes a place we can get to – or a kind of self we can inhabit – when we're more able to feel the pain we've been trying to avoid, through the kind of trauma work described above. We can be less afraid of the feelings that come up when we're triggered because we're more able to expand around them and encompass them when they do. This means that our survival strategies can loosen and our body can relax instead of bracing and contracting. Then we can spend more of our time in the present place, in the centre of the compass. There we're more able to feel whatever feelings arise without being flooded by them. We can be where we are now, rather than carried away in memories of the past or hopes and fears about the future.

Just as there are meditative - and other – practices to cultivate mindfulness when sitting still, and in everyday life, there are practices which we can do, ourselves, to cultivate our capacity to approach sex specifically in such ways.[61]

As we saw in Chapter 3, sex therapists often offer 'sensate focus' techniques where partners take sex off the menu entirely and very gradually engage in sensory practices where the focus is on learning what kind of touch each person enjoys and how to communicate this. The Wheel of Consent community recognises that many of us have no idea how to even tell what sensations we like, let alone how to communicate them with others.[62] They offer the individual practice of 'waking the hands' to gently explore touching an object and tuning in to what feels good to us. This can be followed by the partnered 'three-minute game' which enables people to practise giving and receiving non-sexual touch in ways which are consensual with themselves and others. Through this they learn how to ask to touch or be touched, to agree or refuse, and to engage in ongoing communication.[63]

Expanding the erotic

Reaching a place where we can approach sex – or anything – mindfully, consciously, and consensually is very hard if we have any sense that our bodyminds *should* work in a particular way. We need to open to the possibility that what we'll discover when we tune into ourselves and our desires could be anything, rather than trying to predict and control it, or make it stay the same over time. For example, we need to allow ourselves the freedom to discover that we're not interested in sex at all, that the sex we're interested in differs to the norm, that it doesn't fit the stories we've previously told ourselves and others about our sexuality, and even that we have some disturbing or non-consensual desires. Having conscious awareness of these will make it far less likely we'll unconsciously act out of them and easier to get support around them.

Of course, such openness is incredibly hard in a culture where there are such strong sexual scripts, and stories about what kinds of erotic desires and activities are good and bad, right and wrong, healthy and unhealthy, where maintaining our closest relationships, our vital communities, and our safety in the world are often contingent on having certain kinds of sexual identities, expressions, or experiences.

Black feminist author Audre Lorde reflected that even our equation of 'the erotic' with sex is far too narrow and restrictive.[64] Lorde suggested that we could see the erotic as any experience of being lit up or energised by a kind of life source or power. The erotic connects us to others and to ourselves through passion and vulnerability, deep feeling, and creativity. As well as engaging sensually with a partner, Lorde gives examples of the erotic such as feeling the sun on our skin, writing a poem, building a bookcase, dancing, or passionately engaging in anti-oppression work. She sees the erotic as essential for political action as well as for individual agency and spirituality. The erotic has the power to transform even ordinary things into something deeply fulfilling, making us feel more alive.

There's much to learn here from asexual communities (see Chapter 3). Instead of misunderstanding asexuality as being about restriction (no sex), we could understand it as a refusal to limit our eroticism to one narrow form, with all the problematic assumptions and expectations which go along with this. Asexuality can be a passion for expanding the erotic to include whatever makes us feel most alive.[65] This aligns with many neurodivergent communities where people emphasise the deep pleasure they find in immersing in areas of intense interest.[66]

Like asexuality and the erotic, aromanticism can be seen as a refusal to limit our capacity for *intimacy* to romantic love or partnership. This can highlight the problems which come with restricting love to romantic and familial forms and regarding ourselves and those we love as somehow more valuable than other humans, organisms, and the world we share.

Audre Lorde and other Black feminists, along with many indigenous, disability justice, and spiritual writers, have stressed all of our interconnectedness, interdependence, and interbeing.[67] This is quite different to the separate self of colonialism and capitalism: in competition with others and endeavouring to conquer natural forces. Instead, such perspectives see us as completely entangled with other beings and embedded within wider ecosystems: their surviving and thriving is essential to our own.

Expanding our concept of intimacy beyond our close relationships, and the erotic beyond what brings us individual pleasure, could be a vital part of addressing the separation, disconnection, and polarisation that's at the root of so much human conflict and the ecological crises we face (see Chapter 5). What might it mean to make a lifelong intention of falling in love with the world, regarding all beings as our beloveds? To insist that our own freedom to experience erotic aliveness is contingent on everyone being able to do so?[68]

Many people are now consciously cultivating intimate connections with nature, land, water, plants, and animals in order to reconnect themselves and their communities.[69] This includes ecosexuals who delight in erotic and sensual engagement with the wild and the elements[70] and queer ecologists who explore the potentials in our intimate and erotic connections with the more-than-human world.[71]

Given the role of traumatised/traumatising wider culture in restricting our eroticism and intimacy, such engagements would – perhaps inevitably – take us to a place of seeking social change as well as transforming us at the level of personal experience and relationships.

CONCLUSIONS

It would be wonderful to see psychologists engaging further with the ways cultural – and psychological – understandings of sex might open up our capacities for eroticism and intimacy, instead of closing them down. It would also be great to see more applied psychology on the benefits of becoming more conscious about sex and the mechanisms for doing so, ideally feeding this back into popular culture and into sex and relationships education.

Hopefully this chapter has demonstrated how helpful it would be if we could *all* engage in projects of excavating our unconscious cultural and personal trauma patterns, enabling us to engage with ourselves, others, and the world in more conscious and consensual ways. Returning to the original meaning of psychology as the study of the psyche – perhaps then we might all become psychologists of sex and, indeed, of everything.

NOTES

1 Dabbous, R. (2023). A science of sexuality is still possible — but not in the traditional sense. *The Conversation*, June 13th. Available from: theconversation.com/a-science-of-sexuality-is-still-possible-but-not-in-the-traditional-sense-206979

2 If you're UK based, there's an excellent list of support services here: mind.org.uk/information-support/types-of-mental-health-problems/trauma/useful-contacts. Otherwise an online search should point you towards resources and support for survivors of sexual violence or other forms of trauma.

3 Denman, C. (2017). *Sexuality: A biopsychosocial approach*. Bloomsbury Publishing.

4 See en.wikipedia.org/wiki/Bodymind_(disability_studies) for the origin of this term. I'm using it here to signify how all our psychological and physiological systems are completely interconnected. For

example, our neural pathways wire up and deepen in certain ways, our nervous system is activated in certain ways, our endocrine system cascades certain hormones, our skin becomes more or less sensitive, our senses sharpen or dim, our levels of energy increase or decrease, etc. See Badenoch, B. (2017). *The heart of trauma*. WW Norton & Company.

5 Donovan, C., Gangoli, G., King, H., & Dutt, A. (2023). Understanding gender and sexuality: The hidden curriculum in English schools. *Review of Education, 11* (3), e3440; Horeck, T., Ringrose, J., Milne, B., & Mendes, K. (2024). # MeToo in British schools: Gendered differences in teenagers' awareness of sexual violence. *European Journal of Cultural Studies, 27* (5), 856–875.

6 See Chapter 2 for a reminder of how the bio, psycho, and social are interconnected.

7 In our Jessica Kingsley book *How to Understand Your Sexuality* (2021) Alex Iantaffi and I emphasise the equal importance of pleasure and trauma in shaping our sexualities.

8 Saketopoulou, A. (2023). *Sexuality beyond consent: Risk, race, traumatophilia*. New York University Press.

9 Saketopoulou, A., & Pellegrini, A. (2024). *Gender without identity*. New York University Press.

10 Taxidis, G. (2024). Biopsychosocial – and mysterious! A Queer Jungian perspective on the meaning of GSRD. In D. Davies, S. Neves, & A. Prunas (Eds.), *Gender, sex and relationship diversity therapy: Theory and practice* (pp. 145–155). Routledge.

11 Rubin, G. (1984). Thinking sex: Notes for a radical theory of the politics of sexuality. In C. S. Vance (Ed.), *Pleasure and danger: Exploring female sexuality* (pp. 267–319). Pandora.

12 Haines, S., & Newman, F. (2007). *Healing sex: A mind-body approach to healing sexual trauma*. Cleis Press; Richards, T. N., & Reid, J. A. (2017). Sexual assault and abuse. In A. Vossler, M. J. Barker, G. Pike, & C. Havard, (Eds.), *Mad or bad?: A critical approach to counselling and forensic psychology* (pp. 125–140). Sage.

13 restorativejustice.org.uk/restorative-justice-and-sexual-harm

14 Phillips, N. D. (2016). *Beyond blurred lines: Rape culture in popular media*. Bloomsbury Publishing PLC.

15 O'Neal, E. N. (2019). "Victim is not credible": The influence of rape culture on police perceptions of sexual assault complainants. *Justice*

Quarterly, 36 (1), 127–160; Tosh, J. (2019). *The body and consent in psychology, psychiatry, and medicine: A therapeutic rape culture*. Routledge.

16 Herman, J. L. (2015). *Trauma and recovery: The aftermath of violence--from domestic abuse to political terror*. Hachette UK.

17 Wager, N. (2017). Memory. In *Mad or bad?: A critical approach to counselling and forensic psychology* (pp. 253–266). Sage; Greene, C. (2025). Defendants in sexual assault cases are just as likely to misremember the event as alleged victims. *The Conversation*, August 27th. Available from: theconversation.com/defendants-in-sexual-assault-cases-are-just-as-likely-to-misremember-the-event-as-alleged-victims-new-study-262841.

18 Also called 'modernity': McGee, S., & White, J. (2023). Psychotherapy in modernity a discussion paper for UKCP Member's Forum. Available from: psychotherapy.org.uk/media/bmsdivdv/psychotherapy-in-modernity.pdf.

19 For how these things played out historically, and remain today, see Manjapra, K. (2020). *Colonialism in global perspective*. Cambridge University Press; Butler, J. (2004). *Precarious life: The powers of mourning and violence*. Verso.

20 Arvidsson, H. G., & Visionaries, V. (2025). Blue Horizons: Integrating Marine Ecotourism, Cruise branding, and ocean conservation in the Wake of David Attenborough's Ocean. Available from: researchgate.net/profile/Henrik-Arvidsson-3/publication/392093579_Blue_Horizons_Integrating_Marine_Ecotourism_Cruise_Branding_and_Ocean_Conservation_in_the_Wake_of_David_Attenborough's_Ocean/links/68342ac0026fee1034fbf053/Blue-Horizons-Integrating-Marine-Ecotourism-Cruise-Branding-and-Ocean-Conservation-in-the-Wake-of-David-Attenboroughs-Ocean.pdf.

21 See Chapter 2 on Intersectional Sexualities for more on this.

22 For more on this, see: Barker, M. J., & Iantaffi, A. (2025). *How to understand your relationships: A practical guide*. Jessica Kingsley Publishers; TallBear, K. (2018). Making love and relations beyond settler sex and family. In A. Clarke & D. Haraway (Eds.), *Making kin not population: Reconceiving generations* (pp. 145–164). Prickly Paradigm Press.

23 Hemphill, P. (2025). *What it takes to heal: How transforming ourselves can change the world*. Random House.

24 Shotwell, A. (2016). *Against purity: Living ethically in compromised times*. University of Minnesota Press.

25 Lorde, A. (2018). *The master's tools will never dismantle the master's house.* Penguin classics.

26 Akómoláfé, B. (2025). Becoming sanktuaree. Available from: 986st.r.sp1-brevo.net/mk/mr/sh/SMJz09SDriOHTzlPxjgQEanJwRMr/d1gbt2YEUcfL

27 See Khan, S. (2021). *The roles we play.* Myriad Editions for a beautiful depiction of how historical, cultural, intergenerational, and developmental trauma weave together in shaping experience.

28 Iantaffi, A. (2020). *Gender trauma: Healing cultural, social, and historical gendered trauma.* Jessica Kingsley.

29 This is metaphorical rather than necessarily literal 'holding' and 'hearing'. It's about an adult attuning to a child and finding what's needed in order for them to move through their feelings. Sometimes – for example, with some neurodivergent and disabled kids – it may be important that this *doesn't* involve physical touch or that the child can express themselves non-verbally.

30 Van Der Kolk, B. (2015). *The body keeps the score.* Penguin; Maté, G. (2011). *When the body says no: The cost of hidden stress.* Vintage Canada; Rothschild, B. (2000). *The body remembers: The psychophysiology of trauma & trauma treatment.* WW Norton & Company.

31 Levine, P. A. (2010). *Healing trauma.* SoudsTrue; Kain, K., & Terrell, S. (2018). *Nurturing resilience.* North Atlantic Books.

32 Walker, P. (2013). *Complex PTSD: From surviving to thriving.* Azure Coyote Publishing.

33 Adapted from: Walker, P. (2013). *Complex PTSD: From surviving to thriving.* Azure Coyote Publishing; and Nathanson, D. L. (2014). Affect theory and the compass of shame. In Melvin R. Lansky, Andrew P. Morrison (Eds.) *The widening scope of shame* (pp. 339–354). Routledge. See Dolezal, L., & Gibson, M. (2022). Beyond a trauma-informed approach and towards shame-sensitive practice. *Humanities and Social Sciences Communications,* 9 (1), 1–10.

34 We could connect flight strategies to 'dysfunctional' sex (Chapter 3), given how often this involves trying to repress non-normative desires, perform normative kinds of sex, and make our bodies respond in ways we've been told they should. We could connect the three other strategies more to non-normative kinds of desires (see Chapter 4).

35 There's a guide which takes you through this at: Barker, M.-J., & Hancock, J. (2017). *Understanding ourselves through erotic fantasies*. Available from: patreon.com/c/culturesexrelationships/shop.

36 Lehmiller, J. J. (2018). *Tell me what you want*. Da Capo Press; Lehmiller, J. J., & Gormezano, A. M. (2023). Sexual fantasy research: A contemporary review. *Current Opinion in Psychology, 49*, 101496.

37 A recent example is Anderson, G. (2024). *Want*. Bloomsbury, which takes the classic Nancy Friday collections as a model, as does: Dubberley, E. (2015). *Garden of desires: The evolution of women's sexual fantasies*. Virgin Books.

38 Haines, S. K. (2019). *The politics of trauma: Somatics, healing, and social justice*. North Atlantic Books.

39 For a thoughtful exploration of how we might relate to such fantasies, see Blake, P. (in press). *Unspeakable Fantasies*.

40 Morin, J. (2012). *The erotic mind: Unlocking the inner sources of passion and fulfillment*. HarperCollins.

41 Kahr, B. (2006). *Sex and the Psyche: The untold story of our most secret fantasies taken from the largest ever survey of its kind*. Allen Lane.

42 Barker, M. (2002). *Slashing the slayer: A thematic analysis of homo-erotic Buffy fan fiction*. Presentation to the First Annual Conference on Readings Around Buffy the Vampire Slayer, Blood, Text and Fears, University of East Anglia, Norwich, 19–20 October 2002. Available from: oro.open.ac.uk/23340/2/Barker(1).pdf.

43 Perel, E. (2007). *Mating in captivity: Unlocking erotic intelligence*. Harper.

44 Rowan, J., & Cooper, M. (Eds.) (1998). *The plural self*. Sage.

45 Barker, M.-J. (forthcoming 2026). Incorrigibly plural. In N. Walker (Ed.), *Neuroqueer theory and practice*. Autonomous Press.

46 Fadiman, J., & Gruber, J. (2020). *Your symphony of selves: Discover and understand more of who we are*. Simon and Schuster.

47 See Barker, M.-J. (2023). *Triangles and circles of selves*. Rewriting the Rules. Available from: rewriting-the-rules.com/zines

48 Fern, J., & Cooley, D. (2025). *Transforming the shame triangle*. Thornapple Press.

49 Blinne, K. C. (2012). Auto (erotic) ethnography. *Sexualities*, 15 (8), 953–977.

50 Blake, P. (in press). *Unspeakable Fantasies*.

51 Barker, M. J. (2013). *Mindful counselling & psychotherapy*. Sage; Brotto, L., & Barker, M. (Eds.). (2014). *Mindfulness in sexual and relationship therapy*. Taylor & Francis.

52 Treleaven, D. A. (2018). *Trauma-sensitive mindfulness: Practices for safe and transformative healing*. WW Norton & Company.

53 E.g. Kain, K., & Terrell, S. (2018). *Nurturing resilience*. North Atlantic Books, Shapiro, F. (2001). *Eye movement desensitization and reprocessing (EMDR)*. Guilford Press; trueselftv.com

54 See somaticsexology.school; sexologicalbodyworkers.org/whatis

55 See mind.org.uk/information-support/types-of-mental-health-problems/trauma/treatment-and-support

56 Davies, D. Neves, S., & Prunas, A. (2025). *Gender, sex and relationship diversity therapy*. Taylor & Francis.

57 See Barker, M.-J. (2026). Towards a plural affirmative therapy. In N. Walker & A. Reichart (Eds.), *Neurodiversity in clinical psychology and counseling*. W.W. Norton; ifs-institute.com, powertotheplurals.com/plurality.

58 For example, ACA is a twelve-step programme for people from traumatised/traumatising families: adultchildrenofalcoholics.co.uk; Intentional peer support helps people to form peer support mechanisms: intentionalpeersupport.org; Microsolidarity is a community for forming solidarity groups: microsolidarity.cc.

59 Allen, R. (2021). *Grounded: How connection with nature can improve our mental and physical wellbeing*. Hachette UK; Totton, N. (2021). *Wild therapy*. PCCS Books.

60 For an in-depth exploration of how personal, cultural, and sexual trauma relate to sexuality and sexual difficulties, and what kinds of therapeutic tools can help with this, see Ashton, S. (2025). *Sexual symptoms as trauma responses*. Jessica Kingsley.

61 Barker, M. J. (2013). *Mindful counselling & psychotherapy*. Sage.

62 Martin, B. (2021). *The art of receiving and giving: The wheel of consent*. Luminaire Press; schoolofconsent.org.

63 See artofconsent.co.uk/wheel-of-consent. More on this in: Barker, M. J., & Iantaffi, A. (2025). *How to understand your relationships*. Jessica Kingsley.

64 Lorde, A. (1984). *The uses of the erotic: The erotic as power*. In Sister outsider. Crossing Press.

65 Przybylo, E. (2019). *Asexual erotics: Intimate readings of compulsory sexuality*. The Ohio State University Press.

66 Walker, N. (2021). *Neuroqueer Heresies*. Autonomous Press.

67 E.g. Mingus, M. (2017). *Access intimacy, interdependence and disability justice*. Available from: leavingevidence.wordpress.com/2017/04/12/access-intimacy-interdependence-and-disability-justice. Holst, M. A. (2021). "To be is to inter-be": Thich Nhat Hanh on interdependent arising. *Journal of World Philosophies*, 6(2), 17–30.

68 See brown, a. m. (2019). *Pleasure activism: The politics of feeling good*. AK Press.

69 Macy, J. (2006). *The work that reconnects*. New Society Publishers.

70 Sprinkle, A., & Stephens, B. (2021). Ecosexuality: The story of our love with the Earth. *Ecopoiesis: Eco-Human Theory and Practice*, 2 (1), 42–48.

71 Parkinson, B. (2023). Eco dance movement psychotherapy (EDMP) and queer embodied kinship with the more than human world. *Body, Movement and Dance in Psychotherapy*, 18 (4), 261–274; Taxidis, G. (2024). Living your animal: Listening to wild gender and sexuality. *Psychological Perspectives*, 67 (4), 378–393.

FURTHER RESOURCES

Throughout this book the notes provide suggestions for further reading on each of the topics we've covered. Here are some books and resources that are particularly helpful if you want to find out more about sex and sexuality more broadly.

MY BOOKS

I've written a few other books - with various collaborators - which explore the topics and themes from this book in more depth, or in different ways.

This book is a comic book introduction to sex, which covers some of the same themes as *The Psychology of Sex*, and some other themes as well. There are also graphic guides about gender, and queerness, in this series.

Barker, M. J., & Scheele, J. (2021). *Sexuality: A graphic guide*. Icon Books.

If you want a guidebook for exploring your own sexuality, this should help. There are also companion books on gender and relationships in the trilogy:

Iantaffi, A., & Barker, M.-J. (2021). *How to understand your sexuality*. Jessica Kingsley.

If you want more on how you might apply these ideas to your sex life, this book covers it:

Barker, M. J., & Hancock, J. (2017). *A practical guide to sex*. Icon Books.

This is a self-help style book which applies the kinds of approaches we've taken here to relationships more broadly:

Barker, M.-J. (2026). *Rewriting the rules*. Routledge.

OTHER BOOKS

There are a few useful introductions to sex and sexuality from different starting points which you might find helpful:

For a mainstream psychology textbook on human sexuality, Justin Lehmiller's book is comprehensive and up to date:

Lehmiller, J. J. (2023). *The psychology of human sexuality*. John Wiley & Sons.

For an in depth description of how personal, cultural, and sexual trauma work, and how they relate to sexuality and sexual problems, Sarah Ashton's book for practitioners is excellent:

Ashton, S. (2025). *Sexual symptoms as trauma responses*. Jessica Kingsley.

Two very accessible books on the history of sex and sexuality are:

Lister, K. (2020). *A curious history of sex*. Unbound Publishing.

McCann, C. (2018). *All you need to know... sexuality*. Connel Publishing.

Two short introductions to the sociology of sexuality are:

Mottier, V. (2008). *Sexuality: A very short introduction*. Oxford University Press.

Weeks, J. (2004). *Sexuality: Key ideas*. Routledge.

A short overview of sexology more broadly is:

Neves, S. (2022). *Sexology: The basics*. Routledge.

If you're interested in more on the biopsychosocial approach try:

Denman, C. (2017). *Sexuality: A biopsychosocial approach*. Palgrave Macmillan.

Fausto-Sterling, A. (2012). *Sex/gender: Biology in a social world*. Routledge.

A great book on sex and sexuality from a more global, media studies, perspective is:

Smith, C., & Attwood, F. (Eds.). (2017). *The Routledge companion to media, sex and sexuality*. Routledge.

For a more global approach to sexuality generally, check out:

Davy, Z., Thoreson, R., Bertone, C., & Santos, A. C. (2020). *The SAGE handbook of global sexualities*. Sage.

A wonderful introduction to all things LGBTQIA+ is:

Jeffs, L., & Oakley, S. (2025). *Do ask, do tell: Queer life, love and culture laid bare*. Pan Macmillan.

Jessica Kingsley publishers have many books exploring various sexualities and genders in depth.

uk.jkp.com/collections/all-gender-and-sexuality

OTHER RESOURCES

You can check out my zines and free books on various topics including sex, sexuality, and consent on rewritng-the-rules.com

Justin Lehmiller has a blog covering psychological research on sex and sexuality at lehmiller.com

Psychology Today often includes articles on sex-related topics: psychologytoday.com/gb/basics/sex

At *The Conversation* academics write brief, accessible articles about all kinds of topics. You can access the articles about sex at: theconversation.com/topics/sex

There are many good TED talks about sex and sexuality: ted.com/topics/sex

For more academic papers, the Taylor & Francis journal *Psychology & Sexuality* has a good collection of articles on these topics: tandfonline.com/journals/rpse20

The British Psychological Society has a *Gender, Sexuality and Relationship Diversity Section* section: bps.org.uk/member-networks/gender-sexuality-and-relationship-diversity-section

Pink Therapy is a great organisation for therapists specialising in *Gender, Sex and Relationship Diversity* and publish excellent books on these themes: pinktherapy.com

www.ingramcontent.com/pod-product-compliance
Lightning Source LLC
LaVergne TN
LVHW010838120826
845149LV00017B/3154